JONES

Sensual drugs

Sensual drugs

Deprivation and rehabilitation of the mind

HARDIN B. JONES
Professor of Medical Physics and Physiology
University of California, Berkeley

and HELEN C. JONES

CAMBRIDGE UNIVERSITY PRESS

Cambridge
London   New York   Melbourne

Published by the Syndics of the Cambridge University Press
The Pitt Building, Trumpington Street, Cambridge CB2 1RP
Bentley House, 200 Euston Road, London NW1 2DB
32 East 57th Street, New York, NY 10022, USA
296 Beaconsfield Parade, Middle Park, Melbourne 3206, Australia

First published 1977

Reprinted 1977 (twice)

Printed in the United States of America
Typeset by Bi-Comp, Inc., York, Pennsylvania
Printed and bound by Vail-Ballou Press, Inc.,
Binghamton, New York

Library of Congress Cataloging in Publication Data
Jones, Hardin Blair, 1914-

Sensual drugs.

Bibliography: p.

Includes index.

1. Neuropsychopharmacology. 2.   Drug abuse.
3.   Drugs – Side effects. 4. Sex (Psychology).
I.   Jones, Helen C., joint author. II.   Title.
[DNLM: 1.   Drug abuse. 2.   Drug dependence.
WM270 J764s]
RM315.J55   615'.78   76-8154
ISBN 0 521 21247 2 hard covers
ISBN 0 521 29077 5 paperback

Contents

iii

Foreword

This is a book both for the drug user and for those who have to deal in practice, whether professionally or in ordinary life, with the problems arising from drug use. Dr. Hardin Jones brings to it, not only a long experience of work on the physiology and epidemiology of the health sciences, but also a recent and exceptional experience with two of the most important groups of drug users: the soldier in Vietnam and the university student. Drawing particularly on this knowledge, he and his wife have written a general, readable account of the main drugs in question, of their effects, of the consequences of their chronic use, and of how to help the user. The treatment throughout is integrative; the many lessons common to all the drugs are brought out; the human organism is treated as a whole.

Some of what they say will inevitably be controversial, and because of the extent of multiple drug use and of the very nature of the activity, controlled experimental or epidemiological evidence is not likely soon to come to hand to settle all the issues. A useful feature of their discussion of such issues is that they tackle, not so much the theoretical considerations often raised, but the comments and criticisms derived from their experience with drug users themselves.

Perhaps the most novel and interesting aspect of this book is the stress laid on the impairment in the drug user of the capacity for enjoyment, both generally and of sexual function in particular. While throughout the drug literature, sexual undertones have long been detectable (like a concealed ground bass), here this aspect is taken seriously, broadened, and discussed in a way any drug user can verify for himself.

One hopes very much that the book will be widely read by those involved even if, because it denies so many cherished assertions, it is also attacked. The drug user will find he is regarded, not as a statistic or a patient or a physiological specimen or a psychological deviant or a criminal, but as a person (with all that this implies) who may need help. The ultimate advice offered by Helen and Hardin Jones may seem old-fashioned enough – a resolution to give up drugs; improvement of general health; development of the capacity for enjoyment; support, affection, and reestablishment of self-confidence; and attention to spiritual needs. But it seems more realistic than many programs, and the rational connection between this advice and our knowledge of human physiology is well explained. To my mind, one of the deepest indictments of Western culture is, not the existence of a drug "problem" (that is an ancient phenomenon), but the fact that for many, their use of drugs has been the most interesting thing they have yet met in life. It is because the book takes things seriously at this level that I so willingly write this foreword.

W. D. M. Paton, C.B.E., F.R.S., D.M.
Professor of Pharmacology
University of Oxford
Fellow of Balliol College, Oxford

Preface

As a physiologist, I have done research on the long-term effects of tobacco, alcohol, radiation, and childhood diseases on the human body. My work has been used as evidence of the ways life styles affect patterns of health and disease. This research quite naturally led to an interest in the physiological and psychological effects of psychoactive drugs.

In 1970, I taught a course on drug abuse at the University of California at Berkeley. I have since given the course twelve times, and more than 2,500 students have elected to take it. Many of the students had no background in physiology, and I had to find a way to explain to them the complex effects of drugs. I have used the approach I developed for that course and much information from the lively discussions that followed my lectures in preparing the material for this book.

I have also interviewed more than 1,900 drug users over the past twelve years – students from my classes who came to me for help; GI addicts in the United States, Germany, Thailand, and Vietnam; and young drug users in rehabilitation centers around the world. These interviews have given me much insight into the effects of the psychoactive drugs on the brain. They have also led me to the study of the effects of drugs, particularly heroin, on the sexual processes: the stimulation of sexual sensations, the alteration of sexual responses, and the impairment of sexual functions. The heroin users I talked to substantiated my belief that the drug causes a progressive impairment of these processes.

Over the past few years, I have also studied drug treatment centers around the world and have talked to young drug users of all nationalities about their addiction and rehabilitation. The material gathered on these visits has helped me understand the patterns of drug abuse and the processes and problems of rehabilitation.

Through my conversations with drug addicts, casual users, and nonusers, I have discovered that education is, perhaps, the key both to rehabilitation and to preventing the spread of drug abuse. I have found that when drug users understand the consequences of their actions, they can be persuaded to begin rehabilitation. A knowledge of what they must do to rebuild their debilitated minds and bodies and why they must do it helps them through this difficult period.

In this book, I talk mainly about the male drug user. This is the result of circumstance rather than intention. It seemed that more male than female college students came to me for help, and the army's drug statistics, of course, primarily involved men. However, the interviews I have had with women and the various studies involving them indicate that most of the problems of drug abuse are the same for both men and women.

Marijuana is discussed in the main text, but because of the wide interest in the marijuana problem, the facts about marijuana have been compiled in a separate chapter, Chapter 10. In this chapter the questions most often asked about marijuana are answered, and the damaging effects of marijuana, not only on the brain but also on other parts of the body are discussed.

Most of the appendixes contain statistical and technical information. Appendixes 5 and 6, however, extend the discussions presented in the text; Appendix 8 is a list of expert witnesses, referred to throughout the book, who testified before Senate committees on the physical and psychological effects of cannabis.

This book is based on transcripts of my lectures, on notes of my interviews, and on my drafts of other material related to the text. Because the material was originally in oral form, rough notes, and drafts, it was hardly suited for direct inclusion in the book. My wife, who attended my lectures and joined me in my travels, has worked these transcripts, notes, and drafts into the readable text that follows. She redrafted and reorganized my material; incorporated into it information from the extensive literature on the subject; and converted my tables, notes, and illustrations into narrative. The result of her effort is a text that is clear and free from specialized terms. She has written the book in the first person singular – as if I had been the sole author – because she felt it was based on my teaching and research. This book, however, could never have been written without her help.

Acknowledgment

Grateful acknowledgment is made to my many good friends who have given me the benefit of their research; to Alice Rayner as my research assistant; to Mary Ann Tolmasoff, Nancy Snowden and Alex Grendon for their help in preparing the manuscript; and to the Carthage Foundation and to private individuals who supported my scientific studies on drug abuse.

H.B.J.

June 1976

TO

The addicts and ex-addicts who generously shared with me their experiences in relation to drugs and who were my main source of information on drug abuse and rehabilitation procedures.

CHAPTER 1

Introduction: sensual drug abuse

Mood-altering, sensual drugs are not new to man, but their widespread abuse is. People have faith in drugs and the potential of drugs to release them from pain and make them happy.

In the past thirty years, drugs have been discovered that prevent and cure physical disease and reverse the chemical disturbances that occur in some mental illnesses. Excitement over what drugs can do has led people to believe that any ailment, infective or psychic, can be relieved by taking a pill. At the first sign of nervousness, they reach for tranquilizers; if they feel slightly depressed, they try pep pills. Medical journals now advertise tranquilizers, amphetamines, and other mood-altering drugs; doctors prescribe them; and the public expects miracles from them. In such an atmosphere, it is not surprising that drug abuse has spread.

When people become dependent on drugs to solve their problems, they lose the capacity to deal with life's situations through perseverance, self-discipline, and mental effort. It is now often considered naive to expend energy on solving a problem when there is any easy way out. It is a simple step from "look what drugs do for me when I feel depressed," to "imagine what drugs can do for me when I feel good already."

A distinction must be made, however, between medicine and the sensual drugs; we must not disdain the real and important advances science has made. The history of the medical use of drugs goes back twenty-three centuries to Hippocrates, the Greek physician who is regarded as the father of medicine. He was the first to recognize that a remedy must take into account, not only the symptoms of the disease, but also the constitution and habits of the patient.

His principles have come down to us as the dictum that medicine must specifically suit the disease and the patient. That is, when there is a disorder, only a drug that specifically mitigates that disorder should be used. The drug should also have restorative effects, or it will unbalance healthy functions of the brain and body. The correlative of this principle is that a healthy person cannot benefit from taking a drug. This, too, comes from Hippocrates, who said: "Persons in good health quickly lose their strength by taking purgative medicines."

The distinction between medicines and the sensual drugs is simple. Sensual drugs are those that the body has no need for, but that give the user a strong sense of pleasure. Sensual drugs activate the brain's pleasure centers. We do not know precisely how they do this – whether they stimulate the pleasure centers directly or activate them through chemical mimicry. In this text, I will refer to both possibilities as *stimulation*.

The brain governs sensations, moods, thoughts, and actions, not by a magical process, but by an incredibly complex series of chemically regulated controls. These are easily upset by sensual drugs. This disturbance is apparent in the effect of the sensual drugs on the mechanisms that control pleasure and satisfaction. A drug user's craving for the drug continues, but he feels less and less satisfaction. His brain's pleasure reflexes seem to be weakened by artificial stimulation. In severe addiction, the pleasure mechanisms fail to respond to drug stimulation. The drug then imparts only relative relief from misery and suspends the illness of withdrawal. Information from the senses still reaches the brain, but the brain is unable to evaluate the information and interpret it as pleasurable. In contrast, naturally attained pleasure enlarges the sense of satisfaction and can be repeated indefinitely.

Ultimately, the sensory deprivation of the drug addict manifests itself in a general feeling of physical discomfort and in personality changes. The addict feels depressed and fails to respond either to his environment or to other people. His mental disturbance can be quite similar to paranoia. He cannot discern the source of his problem and looks for the cause in everything but himself. Anything external is suspect; he draws further and further into himself. The addict often feels people are looking at him strangely. One told me he wasn't sure when people smiled at him that they were not really laughing. The addict can even lose his sense of being alive. He feels "dead inside." One rehabilitated heroin addict described his sensory deprivation to me: looking out the window, he said, "The sun is shining, the flowers are in bloom, I know these are signs of a good day, but," pressing his chest, "I don't feel it in here." I have seen addicts habitually press their fingers deep into their arms or legs as if to reassure themselves of their own reality. This craving for lost sensations explains in part the addict's need to continue to seek drug-induced sensations.

Much of the debate over the dangers of specific drugs centers on the question of chemical or psychological addiction. A purely psychological addiction is usually considered controllable through conscious effort. Chemical addiction, on the other hand, is considered less susceptible to mental control. Drugs thought to be *merely* psychologically addictive are considered relatively harmless; those that are chemically addictive are thought to have more serious conse-quences. Actually, there is an inseparable relationship between chemical and psychological addiction, and the two forms coincide when the addictive substance is a pleasure-giving drug.

The sensual drugs give pleasure chemically by stimulating the pleasure centers below the conscious level. The brain produces psychological responses to the chemical stimula-tion of its pleasure mechanisms. The brain's controls then become adjusted so that unmistakable discomfort results if the chemical is not supplied. Thus, chemical and psycho-logical addictions are developed at the same time. Break-ing a chemical addiction may be simple compared with breaking the psychological addiction. In fact, a psychologi-cal need for chemically induced pleasure drives even occa-sional users to repeat drug use.

Sensations aroused by drugs are produced in the same region of the brain as are the sexual sensations. This region, which includes the pleasure centers, is located deep in the center of the brain. Most sensual drugs, by artificially stimulating the brain's pleasure mechanisms, duplicate many of the sexual sensations.

Although drugs may stimulate sexual sensations, they are not true aphrodisiacs. Over a period of time, they are likely to depress sexual sensations and functions. Eventually most sensual drugs cause sensory deprivation. Some sensual drugs may even permanently damage brain cells.

If drugs had as great an effect on the appearance of the body as they do on the function of the brain, there would be little question of their harmfulness and no difficulty in con-vincing people that they should not be used. Unfortunately, it is both difficult and impractical to measure damaged or destroyed cells in the brain, and users of cell-destroying drugs often think they are getting by. They are, however, destroying the reserves they will need in later years when their brain cells die naturally. They may never associate their loss of brain power with drug use; indeed, they will never know how much brain power they could have had.

Reduced effectiveness is difficult for the brain to measure, since drugs affect the very parts of the brain needed for self-evaluation. For instance, I have found that people are more easily convinced that marijuana is dangerous because of its harmful effect on the lungs than because of its potential to damage the brain. The lungs seem to have a greater reality; blackened cell lining can be pictured more easily than brain damage. Perhaps the brain resists considering its own destruction. It is foolish, however, to assume that, because the damage cannot be seen or fully explained, it does not exist.

The brain is the least understood part of the body. Research has been limited because of the brain's size and complexity and because of the hazards involved in examining it – especially while it is functioning. Though we know very little about functions contained in the brain, such as the ability to reason and think abstractly, we know more about functions that correspond to activities of the body, such as seeing and sexual activity. These are more easily researched and explained. In the chapters that follow, I will use these activities to help explain the effects of drugs on the complex functions of the brain.

Drug users defend their drug use and refuse to acknowledge the dangers involved. However, I have found that when scientific facts that correspond to the drug users' own experiences are presented to them, hostility turns to receptiveness. They become interested in knowing about the programming of sexual development in the brain; how the brain's control of sexual functioning and sexual dreaming can be disturbed by drugs; how drugs can cause the brain to make colors appear brighter, sounds clearer, and odors more intense; how drugs distort images and the sense of time.

They learn the causes of drug-induced hallucinations, flashbacks, memory loss, pleasure and pain, and changes in mood. They are usually surprised to learn that these effects occur in the brain and that, though fascinating, they are indications of disturbed brain function.

Although destroyed brain cells cannot be replaced, the brain can, in most cases, adjust and recover from both cell damage and disturbances to its chemical and psychic balance. An addict suffering from sensory deprivation can, with time and a great deal of effort, experience natural pleasure again.

Most people, especially young adults, do not want to harm themselves or impede their development. Drug experimenters have been misled by propaganda for "safe and beneficial" drug experiences; they are almost totally ignorant of the dangers involved. When presented with the facts, most users are willing to stop, and nonusers are more firmly convinced not to experiment. Users who have not yet or only very recently developed dependencies can often end their drug use by themselves. Those who are more heavily involved may need more help.

CHAPTER 2

The brain, the senses, and pleasure

When someone says, "That pleases me," he is usually talking about an object, experience, or thought that is the source of his pleasure; but what do objects, experiences, and thoughts have in common that they are all capable of producing a sense of pleasure? How can someone who says, "I just had a good meal," be as sincere in his pleasure as one who says, "I just had a good idea?" The answer is simple: an object, experience, or thought that gives pleasure is a source only in the sense that it is a stimulus. The common factor is a person's own mind, and it is only in the mind that pleasure can be sensed. The brain is the master control for all sensation and therefore correlates, not only sensory data, but memory, thought, and abstract reason as well – all of which can produce a sense of pleasure. There are varieties and degrees of pleasure, to be sure, but all have their genesis in the brain through the operation of what I call the *pleasure mechanism*.

This mechanism is a process that involves sensory information, control and pleasure centers, memory, association, and reason – all translated by the brain into electrochemical pathways and hookups. When a drug user, for instance, derives pleasure from a drug, he is getting pleasure from his brain's mechanism, which is artificially activated by the drug. When the pleasure mechanism is not allowed to operate on its natural terms – when it is abused by drugs – it begins to fail, so that the pleasurable sensations are weakened. Ultimately they may become imperceptible. The person is then sensually deprived. The mechanisms *can* recover, however, and again become sensitive to the natural sources of stimulation, which can give pleasure without harming the mechanism. Restoration of the pleasure mechanism is the key to rehabilitation from drug abuse.

In spite of its importance, and because of its complexity, the brain is still the least understood part of the body: it is said to be perhaps the most highly organized 3 pounds of matter known in the universe. Its sheer capacity for work belies its weight, and it will be no less a marvel if it is ever explained completely.

Actually, we already know a great deal about the operations of the brain; many discoveries are being made, and much can be inferred. The following is a simplified discussion of the functioning of the brain. It is presented to help the reader understand the action of drugs on the pleasure mechanism and to give some indication of the brain's profound and delicate complexity.

Sensory information

Information concerning both the environment and the body is transmitted via the nervous system to the brain from *sensory receptors*. There are vast numbers of these receptors on nerve endings throughout the body, each adapted to receive a specialized kind of sensation. Although dozens of kinds of receptors have been identified, no one knows exactly how many others there are yet to be identified.

In the head are located the sense organs for sight, hearing, equilibrium, taste, and smell, each of which has receptors for different kinds of sensations. For example, the sense of taste has receptors for salt, sweet, and acid and base; sight has receptors for light intensity and the colors. In the skin are the receptors for warmth, cold, pain, and several kinds of touch and pressure. Located more deeply within the body and the brain itself are receptors that give information about the internal state of the body: muscle and joint tension, joint movement, hunger, thirst, visceral sensations, lack of oxygen, and excess carbon dioxide. Messages from some of the receptors do not reach consciousness. We are never directly aware, for instance, of the working of the specialized receptors that monitor the digestive process, urine production, blood pressure, and the thousands of details of body chemistry.

There are receptors that transmit particular sensations from the erotic areas, just as there are receptors for warmth, pain, and cold in the surface areas of the body. Like other sensory receptors, the receptors from erotic areas have special nerve tracts to the brain. Because of the particular sensations and the special nerve tracts, it is possible to say that sex is actually a separate sense.

Control centers

The sheer quantity of raw sensory information continually coming into the brain from the receptors via the nerve tracts would overwhelm the brain if all of it reached the level of consciousness. However, a system of control centers in the brain refines and interprets the raw information and screens data that are irrelevant or that can be handled below the level of consciousness.

The nerves that carry impulse messages from the sensory receptor up toward consciousness are termed *sensory nerves*. Those that carry impulse commands to act to the muscles, to other parts of the brain, or to glands are termed *motor nerves*. To distinguish the control centers, we call the controls involving sensory information *correlative control centers* and those involving the motor commands *coordination control centers*. The motor commands to act that originate below consciousness are called *involuntary*; those that originate in consciousness are *voluntary*.

About 10 billion (American billion; 10,000,000,000) nerve cells, 90 percent of all the cells of the nervous system, are in the brain. These are organized in a highly compact, elaborate system of intercommunication necessary for brain function. Sensory receptors send their messages to the brain along special nerve tracts by initiating waves (impulses) of electrochemical charges that travel both within nerve cells and across the synaptic gap between nerve cells. Specific chemical action within the cells and at the synaptic gap inhibits or excites message transmission along these pathways. Noradrenaline (norepinephrine), acetylcholine, dopamine, and serotonin (hydroxytryptamine) have been identified as chemicals that transmit impulses within certain brain nerve pathways. To respond, the brain initiates impulses that return along a motor nerve tract to effect an action. Communication within the nervous system is based on so complex and delicate a system of impulses that any chemical change in the brain may distort the entire electrochemical system.

The control centers of the brain are arranged in a complex, integrated, hierarchical system that has evolved over millions of years. Throughout this period, new control centers evolved as each new brain area developed; each newly evolved control center connected to previously existing centers. Thus, in the human brain, the controls are arranged in layers from the most primitive up to the most complex, with each successive layer exercising control over those below. It is not surprising, then, that a multitude of control centers forms links in the brain between the sense organs and consciousness, and between consciousness and voluntary activities of the body.

The control centers themselves work below the level of consciousness as part of the brain's network of nerve cells. The closer they are to the outer portion of the brain, where the conscious element resides, the greater their complexity. One center affects a vast array of other centers. When one is altered, the control centers it regulates are also altered, and the centers they regulate follow suit. Therefore, a small change can have profound effects. This is important in relation to the effects of drugs on the brain (Chapter 3).

The brain is constructed so that the subconscious levels reside in its deepest area, while the conscious levels are located in the outer, upper portions (the gray matter zone). Information coming into the brain via the nerve tracts is passed through the correlative control systems until it reaches the appropriate level of consciousness. As much information as possible is handled below the conscious level to free consciousness from involvement with unnecessary details. In the various control centers on the way to and from the conscious level, information is organized, adjusted, and combined with other incoming or outgoing and stored information. Because the conscious level of the brain has been highly developed, the brain can produce rational thought from sensory information.

Evidence now indicates that there are two separate conscious minds in the brain, one in each hemisphere. Each specializes in different modes of thought. In the right-handed person, the left side of the brain is more concerned with analysis, logic, and verbal expression; the right side, with feelings, intuition, and spatial perception. There is communication back and forth, but the connections between the hemispheres are relatively weak compared with the connections within the hemispheres. The two hemispheres working on the same task may process the same sensory information in distinctly different ways; thus, in producing rational thought, the brain has to incorporate the independent interpretation of sensory information from each hemisphere.

Through the mental processes of memory, association, and reason, and through the billions of electrochemical impulses passed among the various levels of the brain, glandular, muscular, and mental responses are generated. All this happens quickly and automatically: the result is a single fleeting thought and a command to act.

Dramatic evidence of the control center's operations below the conscious level is found in the brain's ability to make deductions from the raw information of each sense. Most research about these sensory controls has employed the sense of sight. Of all the senses, sight is the most sophisticated: a person receives up to 90 percent of all his information about the world through his eyes, and the interpretation of visual data requires fully a tenth of the cerebral cortex. In fact, the retina of the eye is a part of the brain; it and the olfactory receptors are the only points at which the brain receives stimuli directly from outside the body.

There are at least six correlative control centers in the brain that assimilate visual information from the eye and produce a unified image. The brain initially receives very limited data produced in bits and pieces. Bits of information from three areas of each retina enter the brain by different routes and must be coordinated; some receptors in the eye perceive only light intensity; others, just a single color. In spite of these limited data, a person is able to perceive depth, to focus on objects both nearby and far away, to see color in his peripheral vision, to judge distance and direction, to recognize form and movement, and to see objects in a stationary position while his body, head, and eyes are all moving at the same time. These feats are made possible by the correlation of the incoming data and stored information. In other words, a large portion of what a person sees is derived in the brain and has little direct connection with the crude image the eyes see. All this happens with little, if any, thought – unless something goes wrong in the correlative control centers or the receptors. With other senses, as with sight, the accuracy of knowledge about the world depends, not on the senses alone, but on the brain's correlation and interpretation of the sensory information it receives.

Numerous control centers operate even farther below consciousness in the autonomic nervous system, which regulates the internal functions of the entire body. These controls must regulate and balance every minute detail of the body's systems. The autonomic nervous system consists of two divisions: the sympathetic and the parasympathetic nervous systems. Each division is composed of its own system of nerves, which are connected to most of the internal organs and to all the glands.

The two systems of nerve pathways are chemically balanced so that when one is active and dominant, the other is proportionally less active. The two systems work in coordinated opposition: one acts as the accelerator, the other as the brake, to keep body functions in control. Among its other functional duties, the sympathetic system dilates the pupils of the eyes and the bronchioles of the lungs, increases the activity of the heart, raises blood pressure, and inhibits the activity of the smooth muscles of the alimentary canal. The parasympathetic system reverses these actions or produces just the opposite effects. Generally, the sympathetic division dominates the physiological response to excitement, and the parasympathetic division controls the calmer emotions: relaxation, satisfaction, and even worry or depression. The complementary relationship between these two systems can be seen in the excitement of sexual arousal and the satiation that follows; in the restlessness of hunger and the drowsy contentment that comes after a full meal.

By means of these two divisions, the autonomic nervous system can either activate or inhibit the brain's control systems, depending on the needs of the body. The augmenting or inhibiting factor of the control is determined by hormones, particularly the adrenaline of the sympathetic division, which are released into the bloodstream. When the blood's adrenaline content is high, the sympathetic control centers dominate; when it is low, parasympathetic controls dominate.

Dozens of identified hormones and unknown numbers yet to be discovered, along with thousands of enzymes, regulate body functions. These hormones and enzymes are directly or indirectly regulated by divisions of the autonomic nervous system. It is this system that controls growth and metabolism; a few examples are blood coagulation, sexual functions, digestion, blood pressure, water and salt balance, formation of blood cells, and pigmentation.

Nerve center controls and hormone releases are interdependent. For example, stimulation of the sympathetic centers or the action of sympathetic nerves causes the release of adrenaline, which stimulates the sympathetic nerve centers. There is also a relationship between the adrenaline level and the level of other hormones and enzymes in the blood. It is not so much that adrenaline is the master hormone but that the endocrine (hormone-producing) functions of the hypothalamus and pituitary are also influenced by the relationship of the sympathetic and parasympathetic divisions.

The center for the integration of the visceral functions governed by the autonomic nervous system is the hypothalamus. The hypothalamus is the nerve control center for both divisions of the autonomic nervous system and a master endocrine gland that regulates secretions of the pituitary, which, in turn, regulates secretions of other endocrine glands. Thus, both directly and indirectly, the control centers of the autonomic nervous system balance brain and body chemistry through nerve and chemical regulation. This internal control occurs, for instance, when the receptors in the skin feel cold and send messages of the chill to the brain. The hypothalamus acts as a thermostat and directs shivers, goose pimples, and an increase in the heartbeat; it augments production of adrenaline and thyroid hormone through the action of the sympathetic nervous system. Conversely, in response to heat, it can, by means of the parasympathetic system, produce sweating, a slower heartbeat, and dilation of the skin's blood vessels; and it decreases adrenaline and thyroid hormone production. If a person becomes aware of danger, the amount of adrenaline in the sympathetic system is suddenly boosted: he feels excited or angry and is able to act with increased energy.

The chemical source of moods is also found in the autonomic nervous system. It is usually assumed that a euphoric mood, for example, is produced when the nerves of the parasympathetic system activate the hypothalamus. The hypothalamus, in turn, activates the pituitary gland, which secretes adrenocorticotropic hormone. This hormone causes the adrenal gland to secrete cortisone, which, in large amounts, produces euphoria.

Some of the control centers also work below consciousness to regulate the physiological rhythms of the body. Each of us establishes his own cycle of sleeping or eating very early in his life. These habits are patterned partly by the timing and coordination of the internal systems, partly by the senses, and partly by environmental conditioning. We each have our internal schedules for eating, digesting, and becoming hungry. We sleep partly because we are tired and partly because our visual coordination of light and dark determines that sleep should occur in the dark. Physiological rhythms are generally established on a twenty-four-hour schedule, partly because of the light-dark cycle; but even in complete light or complete dark, or when the cycle is longer or shorter, these rhythms are still proportional to the diurnal cycle. We can become aware of the natural rhythms after we have traveled by air across time zones: the diurnal cycle lags for a while until the body's controls can adjust to a new cycle.

The brain's control centers are extremely important in the functioning of the pleasure mechanisms and are the keys to the correlation of all sensory and stored information. Through them the pleasure centers are stimulated and sensations of pleasure reach consciousness.

Pleasure centers

If information the brain receives stimulates the pleasure centers, it gives consciousness the sensation of pleasure. Normally, the pleasure centers are stimulated by sensory information or by thought. Though little is known about exactly how the brain produces pleasurable sensations, an area in the brain has been found in laboratory animals and in humans where pleasurable sensations can be artificially generated.

This area, the *limbic region*, is deep within the brain. It includes the limbic system and related structures (Figures 1 and 2). The limbic region, which constitutes a major portion of the brain in lower animals and is sometimes referred to as the *old* or *visceral brain*, is the area that expanded in humans to become the *thinking brain*. In the most primitive man, this area was the core of the instincts necessary for survival. In modern man, the expanded thinking brain surrounds the limbic region.

The limbic region plays an important part in the central

control of the autonomic nervous system, in visceral and sexual operations, in olfactory and gustatory sensations, in the control of drives, and in the expression of emotions. Experiments indicate that this area is vital for the process of memory storage. Thus, in addition to the pleasure area, many correlative and coordination control centers are located here.

Results of experiments on this portion of the brain have been interesting. In one experiment using laboratory animals, permanent electrodes were implanted in the limbic region of the brain, and the animals were then trained to stimulate this area by activating a lever that caused a mild, nerve-stimulating electrical current to pass between the electrodes. During this training, the animals quickly established a pattern of frequent self-stimulation. Unless stopped, they continued to stimulate themselves until they dropped from exhaustion, and after sleeping they would immediately start pressing the lever. Even if they had been without food and water, they would choose the lever for brain stimulation rather than levers they knew provided food or water. When it became apparent that these newly learned activities would take precedence over all other drives, including the desire for sexual satisfaction, the experimenter concluded that this region was also responsible in some way for sexual response (Olds, 1956).

Experiments with humans have more definitely established this area as a pleasure center for sexual sensations (Heath, 1972*b*). In one experiment, a patient with electrodes placed in various deep and surface sites of the brain chose to push a button attached to an electrode that stimulated the septal region (in the limbic system; see Figure 2). The patient reported arousal and described a compulsion to masturbate. He had feelings of pleasure, alertness, and warm goodwill. During actual sexual intercourse, recordings from this electrode showed patterns of activity dur-

Lobes of the Cerebrum:

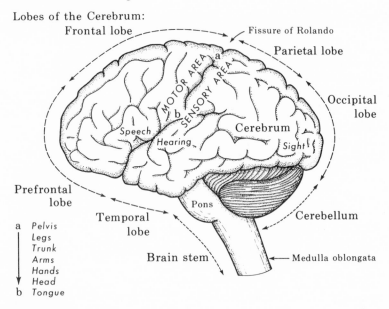

Figure 1. Outer left half, or hemisphere, of the human brain showing major areas controlling conscious sensory and motor functions. From front to back, the brain is divided deeply and symmetrically at the midline into the right and left hemispheres. Sensory and motor functions from each side of the body relate to sensory and motor areas in the opposite hemisphere of the brain. Each hemisphere is subdivided by deep folds of the cerebrum into lobes of specialized functions. Below the joining of the two hemispheres is the brain stem, through which passes all the sensory and motor information between the brain and the nerve trunks – the largest of which is the spinal cord.

ing both preorgasmic and orgasmic stages that did not register in the readings from electrodes in the other areas of the brain. Afterward, except for occasional muscle activity, the readings reflected postorgasmic relaxation.

In another experiment, pleasure-inducing drugs were applied directly to approximately the same region of the brain of a patient. She experienced mild euphoria and awareness that in five to ten minutes culminated in repeti-

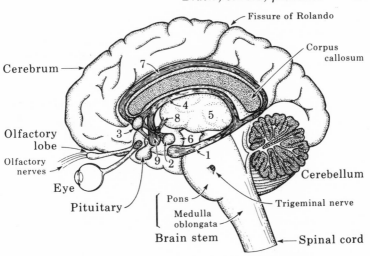

Major structures of the limbic system

1. Hippocampus	4. Fornix	7. Cingulate gyrus
2. Amygdala	5. Thalamus	8. Mammillothalamic tract
3. Septum	6. Hypothalamus	9. Mammillary body

Figure 2. Midplane area of the human brain, viewed from the left, showing major regions of structure and function. Major structures of the limbic system are located in the deepest portion of the human brain. They are arranged in loops of interconnecting nerve trunks and nerve cell clusters. The limbic system controls various emotions and behavioral patterns. The septum contains pleasure centers. The cerebellum is the major control center for motor coordination.

tive orgasms and sensuous movement. Electrode readings showed preorgasmic and orgasmic patterns of activity. Still another patient given pleasure-inducing drugs in the same region said he had never before experienced such intense feelings of pleasure.

It has been established that the limbic region has pleasure areas that are stimulated by sensory information. How many other such pleasure centers there may be is not known. We do know through our own experience, however, that a thought can give us pleasure; it must, therefore, stimulate a pleasure center.

Experimental evidence shows a close relationship between conscious thought and the activity of the limbic region. Memory, association, and certain kinds of thoughts having to do with strong emotions were shown to cause intense brain activity in the limbic region of human subjects. Recordings from electrodes implanted in the region measured a marked increase in activity when the subjects thought of older, emotional memories. For example, activity was registered when one patient recalled his favorite food and when another recalled pleasurable sexual relations. Current thoughts, pleasant or unpleasant, did not always cause activity in the limbic region. An explanation for this is that thoughts that have conditioned the brain's responses for a longer time are the ones most likely to activate the limbic pleasure reflexes. Thus, old stored memories are more likely to produce limbic activity, for more recent ones have not yet conditioned the reflex mechanisms to be associated with the event.

Fortunately, there is no danger that the pleasure centers can be overstimulated by normal sensory information as they can be by drugs or electrical shock, because the body has built-in safeguards for normal, natural stimulation. The sensory correlative control centers, for example, actively depreciate overstimulation of sensory organs: the eye by the variable diameter of the pupil and the variable density of retinal pigments; the ear by the variable conductivity of the bones of the middle ear; the nose by the quantity of air sniffed and by olfactory fatigue. In addition, there are undoubtedly many safeguard mechanisms in the limbic area. Certain parts of the limbic region seem to act as sexual inhibition centers. In a number of subjects destruction of these areas produced an excessive sexual drive that could not be satisfied.

At least some protection from overstimulation comes from the sensory receptors themselves. A London physiologist (H. J. Campbell, 1971) performed extensive experiments in which animals were allowed to engage indefinitely in self-stimulation of peripheral sensory receptors. Some experiments allowed the animals to stimulate themselves with a mild, pleasing shock to the skin; the stimulation caused brain wave responses that were of the same magnitude as the charges naturally developed in the brain by sensory stimulation. Other experiments used a long flash of light for stimulation. The animals stimulated themselves at first at frequent intervals, but the rate gradually declined to zero. Campbell concluded from this experiment that the animals reached satiation because the sensory receptors have the property of *adaptation:* they cease to discharge impulses after a while, even though the stimulation continues. The experimental animals eventually turned to some other activity. The animals who were allowed intracranial self-stimulation, however, never reached satiation; nor did they want anything more than stimulation.

Memory, association, and reason

There are at least three kinds of memory: brief memory (which retains information only for seconds), short-term memory (several minutes), and long-term memory (years). There is also a retrieval process. Short-term memory consists of information some of which is held momentarily and some of which is held for consideration for storage. The information held briefly is easily forgotten, usually within seconds or minutes: a telephone number or the names of people just met. The information that is not lost immediately is sorted out over a period of hours, days, or perhaps weeks, during which time some is lost and some is transferred into long-term memory, to be recalled by degrees. Most information, then, is eliminated during the holding period of short-term memory, and only that which is reinforced by repetition, interest, lack of distraction, or relevance to previous experience is stored in long-term memory. There, it apparently stays for life. One may have difficulty retrieving it, but it is there.

Every memory seems to be stored in a number of different locations; even if much of the brain is destroyed, some memory is still present. It has been speculated that each sense maintains its own memory file from which the correlative control centers draw information to unify the senses. Certain areas, however, have been identified with memory storage. In experiments in which the brains of patients were tickled with low-voltage electrical probes, the patients were able to recall and relive forgotten events in their pasts (Penfield & Perot, 1963).

The area of the hippocampus in the limbic region has been found to be essential for the transfer of information from short-term to long-term memory – essential, that is, for memory storage. When this area is damaged in an accident or in surgery, new information is lost because it cannot be stored (Drachman & Hughes, 1971). A person whose hippocampus has been damaged is still able to recall events that happened a few moments before and events stored in his long-term memory, but not interim events. He is disoriented in time and place and cannot carry on lengthy conversations or make rational connections and decisions. Disturbances in memory storage are often associated with some kinds of brain disorders. The epileptic, for example, does not remember his seizure once he has recovered from it.

Just how memory is stored remains a mystery. The brain's activity is carried on by electrochemical processes (rather than electrophysical processes – in the same sense as electrical circuits – as was once thought), and the memory storage system must be of some related form. The theory of memory is that the information is stored in coded chemical structures such as proteins or nucleic acid (Ungar, 1974). The discovery that nucleic acid (DNA and RNA) synthesis is suppressed in marijuana smokers (Morishima, in U.S. Senate Hearings, 1974) supports this theory, because a prominent effect of marijuana is on the brain's memory systems. One investigator (Pines, 1975) indicates that the transfer of information from one memory stage (short-term, long-term, and others that may be in between) to another may require a chemical process to "fix" the new impression. Other researchers have, in fact, found that hormones produced by the pituitary lengthen short-term memory and aid in the fixation of memory so that information can be permanently stored (Bohus & de Wied, 1966; de Wied & Bohus, 1966).

Studies on the failure of memory have shown that memories are filed in chronological order and apparently layered, with the more recent memories in the top layers. Injuries to the brain, whether by mechanical or chemical trauma, may cause memory disturbances. In such cases, the more recently stored memories are more severely affected. A person with a concussion from a blow on the head, for example, is likely to refer to events of his early life as though they were recent. As he recovers, his oldest memories return first; the most recent, last.

A person who has recovered from a head injury will never remember the few seconds or minutes just prior to the injury, because that information is held so briefly that it is never stored. The same difficulty occurs with the onset of senility. Because those afflicted forget recent events and remember more clearly the incidents of the past, they often seem to return to a second childhood. The senile person may recall events for a few moments, but has trouble storing them in long-term memory. Many kinds of mental illness involve a similar disruption of recent memory, and the inability to connect the present with the past can take the form of mental confusion or hallucination. The disturbed person is able neither to distinguish events according to their importance nor to keep track of their sequence. His memory files become disordered. Such mental confusion and conflict can often cause him to withdraw from the present to live in association with older memories, where his files are more orderly and less destructible.

A good memory is a storehouse of structured and organized information built up by linking new and past information. This storehouse contains not only associated facts and data, but also associated events. With the repetition of sensory information, the mind begins to anticipate recurrence of other events that were associated with that sensory information in the past. Thus, the mind becomes conditioned through repeated associations to expect certain events. At times, when the association is dramatic, a single experience conditions the memory even into its deepest levels. Severe hallucinations such as occur following doses of LSD exhibit this phenomenon.

Short- and long-term memory and associated information are the important tools of reasoning (thought). If these are inadequate, so is reasoning. Conscious thought occurs in the outermost layer (the cerebral cortex) of the brain, but is intricately connected with the levels below, from which it gathers necessary information. The more thought a brain function requires, the more conscious it is. Some memories and associations must be stored just below consciousness (the subconscious), where they can be used with little or no conscious activity or can, when needed, be pulled up to consciousness for use in reasoning.

It is virtually impossible to determine whether certain responses of the body are caused solely by unconscious activity and to assess what proportion of the response is conscious. To illustrate, as discussed before in relation to sight, adjustment of sensory information in the correlative control centers can take place without conscious awareness. Depending on the situation, more conscious activity may be necessary. We have all had the experience of trying to see something in a dimly lit room. As we squint and try to clarify the blurred outline of the object, we construct many possible images of it in our minds. If for a moment the room is brightly lit, we are able to see the object clearly in its true form. After this, if the light is turned out, we are no longer able to conjure up all the possible alternatives for the vague outline before us and can see only the proper image. It appears that a combination of memory, association, and thought goes into the correlative control centers, which then put into the perception a blend of what actually is there and what we expect to be there.

Thought can control voluntary actions. There is evidence that thought can control involuntary actions as well. The latter is sometimes the goal of Yoga and other Eastern meditative religions. Subjects trained in one Eastern technique showed not only an increase in α-wave brain activity (the brain rhythm commonly associated with repose), but changes in other physiological responses as well. The body's oxygen consumption and carbon dioxide elimination decreased even more than during sleep; electrical resistance of the skin, which is usually low during a nervous or tense state, increased markedly during meditation; the heart rate slowed to an average of three beats per minute. Some recent experiments using biofeedback machines indicate that subjects can quickly learn to control blood pressure, heartbeat, and body temperature through conscious effort. It is as if, through concentrated thought, indirect nerve pathways in the brain can be trained to respond or weak nerve pathways are reinforced. The line between voluntary and involuntary acts is not as definite as was once thought.

Not only can thought modify blood pressure, but it has now been established that thought can affect blood flow to the brain. Blood flow to the brain is normally about 50 milliliters of blood per 100 grams of brain per minute. This average value is roughly the same in the few observations that have been made regardless of whether the subject is awake or asleep. Using newer and more refined techniques, Swedish physiologists (Olesen, 1971; Lassen, 1974) have extended the body of information concerning brain blood flow in humans and its relation to thought. They have observed that increased blood flow occurs in that part of the brain responsible for the special mental exertion. For example, the area of the brain responsible for voluntary movement of the hand and arm shows a marked increase in blood flow with vigorous hand exercise. Visual stimulation produces similar focal responses. Mental effort exerted in the performance of simple psychometric tests elicits a moderate increase in cerebral blood flow in wider, but corresponding, regions of the brain. An increase in blood flow is interpreted as providing an increase in food and oxygen for the brain's energy consumption. The theory that thought keeps the mind active and alert now has a physiological as well as a psychological basis.

Awareness of pleasure

The most essential part of the pleasure mechanism is the awareness of pleasure. When sensations of pleasure come to consciousness from the pleasure areas, some of these sensations involve more conscious brain activity than others. The brain activities that can be called *sensation* range from the simplest sensory perception to the most complex emotional states. For this reason, I classify sensations as either primary or derived. The *primary sensations* are those communicated to the brain from the sense receptors with minimal adjustment before reaching consciousness – for example, pain, warmth, cold, touch, taste, odor, movement, light, sound, and some sexual sensations. *Derived sensations* may be a combination of primary sensations or those in which sensory information has been thoroughly linked to associations, memories, and thought – for example, well-being, loss of inhibition, euphoria, calmness or excitement, and exhilaration. The derived sensations are usually closely related to mood.

How primary and derived sensations or moods reach awareness can only be speculated. Communications within the brain are evidently made through linkages of nerve cells. These linkages form pathways through the brain that are either dominant or weak. In a mood, for example, all emotional responses of an individual tend to be similar; events otherwise neutral become colored according to the mood; if one is in a "bad mood," experiences that should bring pleasure do not seem to link up in the brain to register as pleasurable. It is as though pathways through the brain are linked up to make it difficult for other emotions or sensations to break through to consciousness. Mental illness also demonstrates the apparent dominance or weakness of certain thought pathways.

There is increasing scientific evidence that body chemicals play an important role in brain cell communication. The research on mental illness and defects in the orderly transmission of signals across the junctions between the nerve cells in the brain adds to our understanding of brain cell communication. There is now considerable evidence that certain hormones play a key role in transmitting or blocking signals at the junctions of the brain cells.

The modern position is that the brain's communication

system is chemically directed; that chemicals reinforce or weaken the action in each of the brain's individual nerve pathways and direct the hookups between pathways. There are many alternate routes through an untold number of possible hookups to a particular destination in the brain. In a particular mood, for example, some pathways through the brain are reinforced while others become correspondingly weak. When the mood changes, so do the hookups and the dominance of the pathways. It is almost as if one changed heads or switched to different systems and controls inside the head.

The linkages in the brain between the pleasure centers, thought formation, and sensations are, I believe, chemically directed. Therefore, the use of the sensual drugs temporarily reinforces or weakens linkage of the pathways and stimulates or diminishes a sensation. As the brain becomes dependent on drug chemistry for stimulation of the pleasure mechanism, the normal linkages are bypassed; they weaken, and eventually they fail.

CHAPTER 3

Action of sensual drugs

The pleasure mechanism, as defined in Chapter 2, involves sensory input, control centers, pleasure centers, consciousness, memory, association, and reason. The essence of the mechanism is nerve action and chemistry; because it includes so many areas of the brain, we can experience many varieties and levels of pleasure.

In the broadest sense, drugs are taken for pleasure; even in medical practice, they are used to make the patient feel better or "feel good." The problem is to determine when drugs may be used safely to restore mental and physical health and when drug taking becomes abusive and dangerous to health. The healthy body maintains its balance by means of the brain controls, which keep all functions operating smoothly and within the optimal range. Disease throws the body's chemistry outside that range. It is as though the chemicals of the body are on balance scales. Disease overloads one side of the scales (or lightens the load of one side) so that the two measures are unbalanced. When this imbalance occurs, symptoms of the disease appear in such forms as high temperature, increased blood pressure, dizziness, depression, or fatigue. Drugs are administered to put the scales back in equilibrium until the brain's controls are again able to maintain the balance. In some cases, drugs

29

must substitute for a chemical imbalance and, therefore, must be taken indefinitely. There are drugs that can slow or speed the heartbeat, increase or decrease blood pressure or muscular contraction, raise or lower body temperature, clot or liquefy blood, control fluids and secretions, increase or decrease growth, sedate or arouse, or alter mood.

Unfortunately, no drug has yet been found that is absolutely selective in its effects. A doctor has to weigh the effects of the disease against the side effects of the drug. A drug can never precisely duplicate natural controls; drugs act at more than one site, and every site of action is synchronized with other functions that are also slightly altered by a drug.

There is greater danger when drugs are taken by a healthy individual. Picture again the balanced scales of the healthy person: when he takes a drug, instead of being put in balance for the correction of a functional disturbance, the scales are thrown out of balance. Nevertheless, in the desire for immediate gratification and pleasure, people have found that certain drugs, when taken in large enough doses, have sensual or mood-altering effects. Users of such drugs are either willing to risk throwing their controls out of balance or are not aware of the risks involved.

Drugs from plant sources have been used for their sensual and mood-altering effects for hundreds, even thousands, of years. The most widely known are opium, alcohol, cannabis (hashish and marijuana), cocaine (from the coca plant), mescaline (from a Mexican cactus), and various drugs from funguses. Other drugs have been developed through the modification of the chemical structure of natural drugs or through the synthesis of compounds of related structures. LSD (lysergic acid diethylamide) and heroin, for example, are modified drugs – LSD from ergot and heroin from morphine, the principal ingredient of opium. The amphetamines, on the other hand, are synthetics closely related to the naturally occurring drugs cocaine and ephedrine. All these drugs have profound effects on the sensory correlative control centers and the autonomic nervous system.

The same drug can be employed both as a medicine and for its sensual effects. I will use the word *drug* to indicate the latter use and *medicine* to indicate the former. Drugs can be classified according to their chemical structure or their physiological or psychological effects. Because we are interested in the sensual effects of drugs, we will classify them as stimulants, depressants, intoxicants, or hallucinogens, as indicated below:

Stimulants: amphetamines, cocaine
Depressants (major): opiates
Intoxicants (minor depressants): alcohol, barbiturates, tranquilizers, volatile solvents (ether, lacquer thinner, solvents in plastic glues, petroleum fluids, and propellants in spray cans)
Hallucinogens: LSD-25, mescaline, psilocybin, marijuana

The ways these drugs enter the brain, produce sensual or mood-altering effects, and finally impair the pleasure mechanisms are the primary concerns of this and the following chapters.

Many drugs cause some degree of hallucination. We classify as hallucinogens those whose primary effect is faulty processing of sensory information. Marijuana, a mild hallucinogen, and LSD (lysergic acid diethylamide), a powerful hallucinogen, are discussed in this text as typical of these drugs. There are a number of powerful hallucinogens besides LSD: DMT (dimethyltryptamine), DET (diethyltryptamine), STP or DOM (2,5-dimethyl-4-methylamphetamine), DOET (2,5-dimethoxy-4-ethylamphetamine), psilocybin (from a tropical mushroom), mescaline, and others. The forms of visual hallucinations seem similar with each of the powerful hallucinogens; most users cannot tell the difference between them. (In treatment, however, the difference between the hallucinogens may be critical. See Hallucinogens, Chapter 8.)

Cannabis refers to all the psychoactive drugs made from the hemp plant, *Cannabis sativa*. The principal psychoactive ingredient in cannabis drugs, tetrahydrocannabinol (THC), is found in the resin of the flowers and leaves. The strain of the plant, the conditions under which it is grown, and the part of the plant used determine the THC content of the drug derived from it. A few of the terms used for various psychoactive cannabis preparations are *bhang*, *ganja*, *charas*, *kif*, *pot*, *cannabis oil*, *hashish*, and *marijuana*. Marijuana (sometimes spelled marihuana), the Mexican name for a preparation made from the dried flowery tops and leaves of the hemp plant, is the most commonly used form of cannabis in the United States, but hashish, a concentrated form of the resin from the flowers and leaves, and cannabis oil are becoming more available. Hashish is usually, but not always, stronger than marijuana. Both range widely in THC content. Because marijuana is the most common cannabis drug in the United States, the terms cannabis and marijuana are popularly used synonymously when referring to the psychoactive cannabis drugs. I will use the term *marijuana* when referring to psychoactive cannabis preparations except where a distinction seems appropriate or when the literature cited specifically uses another term.

How drugs enter the brain

Like all other parts of the body, the brain is fed by substances carried in the bloodstream and absorbed into the brain through blood vessel walls. Molecules of sugars, oxygen, salts, amino acids, vitamins, and water transported by the blood are passed in this way to the brain tissue. Brain capillary walls are composed of tightly packed cells lacking open pores. Many molecules that could alter functions of the brain are kept from direct contact with it by these special capillaries walls. These walls, called the *blood-brain barrier*, are unique to the brain. They regulate the rate at which molecules enter and leave the brain: small molecules can pass quickly through the blood-brain barrier; larger molecules pass in and out more slowly.

The brain does not store energy and is unable to generate energy in the absence of oxygen. It depends on a constant supply of food and oxygen carried to it in the blood; if it is denied blood for fifteen seconds, loss of consciousness results. If the interruption lasts four to ten minutes, the brain cells are progressively and irreversibly damaged, especially those necessary for thought processes. In contrast, other body cells can live for hours without blood. To keep a constant supply of the substances necessary for the high energy consumption of the brain, a tremendous proportional volume of blood must circulate there. The capillaries in the brain are so small and so numerous that if placed end to end they would measure about 100 miles, but at any one moment they would contain less than 1 teaspoon of blood. Brain activity requires between 10 and 13 percent of the blood pumped by the heart every minute. In other words, a volume of blood equal to the volume of the brain itself must flow through the brain's capillaries every two minutes.

Whether a drug is sniffed, swallowed, smoked, rubbed on the body, or injected, if absorbed it travels through the bloodstream and reaches the brain. The ability of a drug to enter the brain depends on the structure of the blood-brain barrier, the rate of blood flow through the brain, and the special properties of the drug. Because sensual drugs have a low molecular weight, are fairly stable, and are soluble in blood and the fats of cell surfaces, they pass as easily into the brain as sugars, salts, vitamins, and amino acids; and because of the tremendous flow of blood through the brain, drugs can enter different areas of the brain very quickly.

Some areas of the brain are more accessible to drugs than others, largely because of a higher concentration of open capillaries. The cerebral cortex (outer layer of the cerebrum) and the deep brain area, which contains the limbic region, are particularly accessible because they are rich in brain cells well supplied with capillaries. Patterns of blood flow in different parts of the brain also vary with changes in mental state.

(The nerve cell bodies are gray in color, and areas containing high concentrations of nerve cell bodies are called gray matter areas. Although the cerebral cortex is popularly known as the gray matter zone, clusters of gray matter are also concentrated in the deep brain area. Because, as discussed above, the brain nerve cells critically depend on the blood supply for food and oxygen, it is the gray matter in the brain that has the highest capillary content and the highest rate of blood flow – and is the most accessible to sensual drugs.)

Areas of drug action

Drugs travel throughout the circulatory system and pass through blood vessel walls into the organs and tissues. Where they actually have an effect depends both on the circulatory patterns and on the cell chemistry of a particular area.

Drugs reach all the sensory organs (eye, inner ear, taste buds, and touch organs), but the sensory functions of these organs are not necessarily affected; rather, the alteration in these senses is usually caused by an alteration of the brain's sensory-information-control centers. Most drugs accumulate in the liver, kidneys, and intestines because of the high blood flow through these areas. The liver tends to remove the drug along with food fuels by metabolic burning. The kidneys, intestines (aided by bile from the liver), and sweat glands remove the drug from the body through excretion. This is why, incidentally, traces of most drugs are detectable in the urine by sufficiently sensitive tests.

Some sensual drugs can selectively relax or stimulate contraction of the involuntary muscles, especially in the blood vessels, the intestines, or the uterus. The chemical basis of these effects is similar to that in the brain and nerve cells, and it is often difficult to know whether a change caused by a drug is due to action initiated through nerve controls of the brain or to direct action on the involuntary muscles.

Sensual drugs enter the brain quickly and directly or indirectly stimulate the pleasure centers. Capillary patterns and blood flow in the brain and the high susceptibility of brain cells to chemical alteration make the brain largely defenseless against such chemicals.

The limbic region of the brain is particularly sensitive to the sensual drugs; the stimulation of this area produces a multitude of sensations. Little is known about the chemistry of drug action in this region, but because of its dense capillary patterns, this area probably admits the sensual drugs quickly. Chemically regulated control functions, which are concentrated in the limbic region, are then impaired, and the effect spreads to other parts of the brain.

Although many of the primary sensory correlative control centers are located outside the limbic region, the known effects in this area are sufficient to account for most of the drug-induced disturbances of the senses. Even the effects of drugs on reason can be related to controls in the limbic region. The sensual drugs in general, then, seem to affect the subconscious part of the brain. There are a few exceptions, however. The barbiturates, alcohol, tranquilizers, and volatile solvents seem to affect primarily the conscious areas and have secondary effects on the subconscious.

Drugs and the control centers

The widespread effects of a drug on both the brain and the body can be attributed to its action on the cluster of controls for glands and organs within the stalk of the brain that act as relays between the brain and body functions. Even when a drug affects only one control center directly, all the control centers that rely on that one must also alter their activity to some extent; and the controls below those then must also change.

In estimating drug action on the brain's controls, we must start with what we know to be causes and effects. For example, we know through observation and experimentation that alteration of pupil size is caused by the action of the autonomic nervous system's pupillary controls in the midbrain and related areas of the stalk of the brain. Dilation is caused by stimulation of sympathetic nerves or by inhibition of the parasympathetic nerves (this is the effect of atropine, also known as belladonna). Constriction is caused either by inhibition of the sympathetic centers or by stimulation of the parasympathetic centers. We know that a rise in carbon dioxide in the blood initiates signals in the carotid artery that are passed through sensory autonomic nerves to the control centers in the hypothalamus – all of which results in an increase in the breathing rate. The autonomic nervous system is directed from centers in the hypothalamus to muscle coordination centers so that dozens of muscles contract in unison to increase the depth and frequency of breathing.

We also know that a rise in blood pressure and pulse rate is due to an order from the hypothalamus to the small arteries in the body to constrict and also to hypothalamic stimulation of the adrenal glands, which raise the amount of adrenaline in the blood. The increase in sweat and decrease in blood flow caused by anxiety also originate in the autonomic nerve centers of the hypothalamus. Functionally, these controls are able to regulate cooling of the skin; they also reflect the extent to which the thinking brain can influence the autonomic nervous system.

Drugs alter the normal stimulus and response relationships of the autonomic nervous system controls. Exactly how they alter them is, unfortunately, not completely understood. Possibly they amplify natural brain action by mimicking brain chemistry. Possibly their toxic effect alters brain chemistry; that is, drug effects may be a form of poisoning, since all psychoactive drugs, taken in large doses or frequently for a long time, appear to produce toxic changes in the brain that are detectable on microscopic examination. In either case, the chemistry of the nerve transmitter both within and between brain cells is altered or there is a change in the secretion of the many hormones of the hypothalamus and pituitary gland, which in turn alters the controls for the secretion of enzymes and hormones in all parts of the body. Recent experiments performed on animals (Collier *et al.*, 1972) indicate that several neurotransmitter hormones are disturbed by sensual drugs. When the nerve transmitter chemistry in the brain is altered, the abnormal inhibitor/excitor action at the nerve cell junctions either augments or weakens certain pathways through the brain and changes normal functions throughout the brain. For example, many of the brain's controls and pathways are thrown out of balance by a drug such as heroin. Breathing and pulse rate slow; blood pressure is reduced; blood sugar levels are altered; urine excretion is increased; intestines have less movement; biliary and urinary tract sphincters are less responsive; body temperature is lowered; the eyes become red, the pupils constrict, the eyelids droop, and vision becomes less acute; the release of pituitary hormones is decreased; sweating may occur; pain is not bothersome; the mind clouds. An addict after dosing may become suddenly active, then inactive and sleepy. With continued use, constipation and impotence are usual complications. When an addict cannot get the drug, his brain's control centers try to get back in balance. During the period of readjustment, he is hypersensitive, restless, and irritable; his eyes water, mucus runs from his nose, and he yawns persistently. His muscles twitch violently and his back and legs ache severely. All this is accompanied by pains in the stomach, vomiting, and diarrhea. Even in the hottest weather he may feel cold; he itches, and sleep is almost impossible. These conditions continue until his brain's controls can get back in balance.

Drugs and the sensory correlative control centers

The majority of the sensual drugs, the hallucinogens in particular, upset the chemical balance of the communication and response mechanisms in the brain. Sensory information received by the consciousness is distorted in the correlative control centers. The disruption of the correlative control centers below the conscious level produces unreal and distorted images, intensifies or dulls sounds and odors, upsets the sense of equilibrium, intensifies or numbs the sense of touch, and confuses the information to the point of synesthesia: colors are heard or smelled and sound is seen.

We know very little about the complicated process by which sensory information is adjusted from its raw state to an impression the mind finally recognizes. A good example, however, of the illusions caused by the disturbance of sensory correlative control centers is the effect of hallucinogens on the sense of sight. Marijuana smokers often report that when they are high, colors seem to be more vivid than usual. The apparent cause of this phenomenon is the disturbance of visual correlative control centers. We believe that normally we see the entire scope of vision in color; in fact, we see only two small spots directly ahead in full color and the rest in incomplete color muted toward gray at the periphery. By cupping the fingers into a tunnel and holding them against each eye, we can get a rough idea of the portion of vision that is seen in full color. We know that the visual input passes through the correlative control centers of the brain, where a perfect or nearly perfect color image is reconstructed from the immediate data by the scanning of the eyes and by short-term memory. These correlative control centers can also correct for such visual defects as position, focus, or astigmatism, provided each eye has a different defect. The brain thus defies the laws of optics by constructing a better image than either eye can see alone. Marijuana and the stronger hallucinogens alter the mechanisms of color perception, but do not precisely intensify the color. Instead, the phenomenon occurs because the peripheral field of vision becomes fainter under the influence of the drug, and a kind of tunnel vision is produced by dimming the gray side or lateral areas so that the colors in the center of the field seem more intense by contrast.

Most evidence of drug effect on control centers comes from reports of dizziness or giddiness experienced by many drug users. If we were to compare our eyes with a camera, we would expect the vision received by the brain from such a small pair of cameras to be like the tossing image photographed by a hand-held movie camera, since the eyes themselves, the head, and the body are all moving. The fact is, however, that we perceive the world to be stable. The correlative control centers are able to determine the necessary details from the sweep of vision and assemble them in a stabilized image that is then relayed to the consciousness. Sometimes, however, this mechanism breaks down. When motion is random and extreme, the limits for correction are exceeded and we develop motion sickness; if the correlative control centers become fatigued, damaged, or drugged, the image in motion gets through to the level of consciousness. Then, motion rather than the object in view dominates attention. The resulting sensation is giddiness or dizziness, and the person affected often experiences the general discomfort and nausea characteristic of motion sickness. Motion sickness can, of course, also be felt with the eyes closed because several other senses contribute to motion sense and equilibrium, and they too can become fatigued.

Hallucinogenic drugs can disturb vision by distortion of perception when they cause mental pictures from the memory to be projected into present visual images. Some marijuana users interviewed while high have seen friends or familiar objects that were not in the room at all. This form of hallucination is even more pronounced in individuals who have taken LSD, and it shows how easily memory, association, and imagination can distort the sense of vision if the correlative control centers are thrown out of balance. Less frequently hallucinations, particularly those associated with marijuana use, take the form of deletions or additions in a small segment of the field of vision so that the person affected does not notice the difference. This can cause trouble: one marijuana user, on the occasion of his first high, reported: "Driving home on the freeway, I turned off on the Park Boulevard turnoff, except that it wasn't there."

Hearing, equilibrium, taste, touch, and all the other senses can be equally devastated in their correlative control centers. Because the functions of all the senses are interrelated in the brain, a chemical upset in one is likely to affect the others. The distorted information is given to the memory to store for the higher level of the brain to use in processes of association and reasoning. A drug affects some senses more intensely than others. The strong hallucinogens may have such an impact on the correlative control centers that the effect may be likened to a severe mental storm, perhaps interpreted as pleasurable, though very often as frightening.

Drugs and memory

The symptoms of memory loss from whatever cause are difficulty in concentration, absent-mindedness, distraction, mistakes in calculation, inconsistencies, and failure of sequence retention. All these symptoms, from simple absent-mindedness to complete anmesia, can result from a blow on the head, convulsions, shock, or the onset of senility. A number of drugs can produce similar symptoms by a chemical alteration of the memory storage faculties.

Little is known about how memory is stored and transferred from short-term to long-term memory, but the evidence strongly suggests the process is a chemical one, which can be upset chemically. We know, for example, that the powerful sedative chlorpromazine can suppress delirium in persons excited by hallucinogenic drugs or other mental agitation. It decreases short-term memory and memory recall significantly during the several hours of its effect. The hypnotic drug, scopolamine, produces nearly total amnesia for the period of its effect, even though the patient does not lose consciousness.

The sensual drugs can impair memory in a variety of ways. In alcoholic and barbiturate drunkenness, the failure of short-term memory is particularly noticeable. The intoxicated person may have no recollection of the time he was intoxicated, just as the epileptic has no recollection of his seizure, simply because of the temporary blockage of information transfer from short-term to long-term memory.

Marijuana and heroin also depress short-term memory and inhibit the transfer of information to long-term memory so that sequences of time and thought cannot be held in the mind.

Memory registration, retention, and recall are sometimes tested by having a subject repeat sequences of numbers over a period of time. In experiments with tetrahydrocannabinol (THC, the active ingredient in marijuana), subjects given both short- and long-term memory tests show a significant impairment of short-term memory. There is both a failure to recall information and an increasingly inaccurate recall. Short-term memory loss is often seen in a marijuana user's inability to remember in midsentence what he was about to say. One researcher (Huot, 1976) suggests that loss of memory from marijuana use may be related to an action of THC on RNA or protein synthesis (see Chapter 10).

In addition, some drugs cause a complete scrambling of both short- and long-term memory. The sequence of events in time is therefore lost. This often occurs when erroneous sensory information has been stored in the memory and then is integrated with other past memories or with immediate events lodged in the short-term memory.

A more severe form of memory impairment is the flashback. Hallucinations (regardless of the drug inducing them), especially when severe, tend to be followed later by flashbacks, even when no more of the drug is taken. A memory disorder seems to be involved. The confusion of a flashback is like that which occurs when an event triggers memory and we recall a dream: for a moment, at least, the distinction between reality and the dream is blurred. If a person fixes on a single idea, for example, during intense hallucinations caused by LSD, the idea seems to become impressed in the deep, long-term layers of his memory, and no rational argument is sufficient to uproot it.

Some people report that hallucinations have enabled

them to go farther back into their memories and freely associate events of their earlier lives. This may be true, but
what enables them to do this is not a sharpening of long-
term memory, but a dimming of recently stored memory
and recent recall. The effect of the drug brings about a
condition more like senility. The drug taker falls back into
the deeper memory files and behaves, as many observers of
the drug scene report, more immaturely. He probably has
to rely on the deeper levels of memory and patterns of
behavior associated with his childhood.

The disturbances of the memory process are probably
partly related to the drug's effects on sense perception and
other mental functions: the decrease or increase in sensory
images coming into the mind, the distortion of time, the
confusion of time sequences, hallucinations, altered attention span, the inability to pay attention to events in order of
their importance, lack of motivation, the disturbances of
the nerve cell network, and the alteration of chemical coding for new information. Disturbances of short-term memory may be linked to disturbances in the limbic region,
where certain vital processes of memory storage are initiated, particularly the processes through which information
is transferred from short-term to long-term memory.

Stimulants, depressants, intoxicants, and hallucinogens

Since many areas of the brain are affected by a sensual
drug, multiple effects are to be expected, but one or more of
the effects usually dominates the others. There are so many
variables, however, that any classification according to effects is somewhat arbitrary and imprecise.

In general, the stimulants (uppers) and hallucinogens, including marijuana, exert their major mind-altering effects
on regulative centers below consciousness in the autonomic

nervous system and the correlative control centers and have less effect on the conscious processes. The primary action of the stimulant drugs (amphetamines and cocaine) is to increase sympathetic nerve functions, causing blood pressure and pulse rate to increase and the whole body to rise to a higher level of excitement.

We divide the depressants (downers) into two groups: the major depressants and the intoxicants (minor depressants). The major depressants are the opiates. Like the stimulants, their primary mind-altering effects are on the controls below consciousness. They stimulate or mimic the action of the parasympathetic division of the autonomic nervous system, causing a general slowing of the body's responses. The intoxicants (minor depressants) are alcohol, the barbiturates, the minor tranquilizers, and the volatile solvents. These depress the conscious activities of the brain and appear to have less effect on the regulative centers of the autonomic nervous system than do the depressants. Therefore, it is more accurate for this discussion to classify these drugs as intoxicants than as depressants, since this classification acknowledges their effects on the conscious process. The intoxicants also affect motor coordination, possibly because in addition to direct effects, an impaired consciousness gives inaccurate commands to the motor coordination centers.

The hallucinogens, although usually mild stimulants, act primarily on the sensory correlative control centers and on memory. LSD-25, psilocybin, and mescaline are powerful hallucinogens. Marijuana, although sometimes classified as a hallucinogen, is unique among the sensual drugs in that it has different chemical properties from the others and has multiple effects. Marijuana can act primarily as a hallucinogen, a stimulant, a depressant, or an intoxicant, and sometimes as a combination of all four.

Variation in drug effects

Drug effects vary greatly according to dose. Drugs that act selectively on cell enzymes at a low dose may paralyze nerve action at higher doses. A high dose also tends to affect more areas and levels of brain function than does a small dose. Low doses of all the sensual drugs produce euphoria; higher doses bring on more intensely pleasurable sensations. Not only does the intensity of the sensations differ with varying doses, but the type of sensation varies as well. Amphetamines and cocaine, for example, at high doses produce hallucinations. The kinds of sensations induced by marijuana vary markedly with dose: low doses may cause anxiousness, restlessness, euphoria, drowsiness, or disorientation in time; medium doses cause stimulation and talkativeness; higher doses are hallucinogenic; and very high doses incapacitate cognitive and motor functions. The variation in sensations from different amounts of alcohol is well known. Small amounts of alcohol cause feelings of bodily warmth, relaxation, and well-being; medium doses slow mental processes, diminish inhibitions and judgment, and promote drowsiness; high doses produce hallucinations, slurred speech, dizziness, nausea, vomiting, lack of coordination, numbing of the skin, and in some, hostility and rage; very high doses cause unconsciousness and may depress the vital functions enough to result in death.

Drugs taken simultaneously may produce different effects than each would if it had been taken separately. Alcohol and such drugs as barbiturates, aspirin, and chloral hydrate may be ingested safely if taken separately and at widely spaced intervals, but if alcohol is taken in combination with one of these, the effects are intensified and even a so-called safe dose is occasionally lethal. Apparently the brain is able to handle a certain amount of adjustment in its control centers, but there is a point beyond which it cannot keep drug action under control.

The effect of a drug also varies from individual to individual and from time to time. Occasionally, the same drug can even produce entirely opposite effects. For example, most heroin addicts become constipated; a few, however, find the drug has the opposite effect, and they get diarrhea instead. Amphetamines produce feelings of hyperalertness in most people, but a few experience drowsiness; marijuana usually increases appetite, but in some users, appetite is markedly decreased. What causes these individual differences in a drug's effects is not known fully. Some such differences seem to be due to capillary patterns and some to cell chemistry. We also know that the effects vary according to the conditions under which the drug is taken and according to the mood of the individual. We know, for example, that the blood flow in the limbic region of an excited animal can increase many times. We infer from this that in human moods of excitement more of a drug is allowed to reach the limbic region. When the animal is frightened, on the other hand, there is less response to depressant drugs. Experiments with cats, for example, have shown that they cannot be anesthetized when they are frightened. Anesthesia has greater effect in humans too when the parasympathetic nervous system's controls are dominant and they are calm. Anesthetics, depressants, and intoxicants have less effect on an excited person whose sympathetic controls are dominant. Cold water or strong coffee sobers a drunk by generating sympathetic nerve activity and adrenaline production, which wakens his systems, in a sense, and makes him more alert.

Mood-altering drugs

The sensual drugs are often called mood-altering drugs, and though the term is vague, it refers to the fact that when a drug alters sensory information, it also alters the brain's interpretation of that information. In general, a mood is an attitude through which we interpret both the feelings of the body and the circumstances surrounding us. While we can experience several sensations at one time, mood is a predominating state of mind or feeling that lasts over a period of time.

I maintain, as stated earlier, that our awareness of sensation and mood is the result of chemical change in the brain's nerve hookups and of the dominance of certain nerve pathways. That a drug alters the hormonal balance of these hookups and pathways seems to be a major factor in its ability to alter mood. Dramatic changes occur when hormones natural to the body are administered artificially. For example, cortisone can induce a state of euphoria and adrenaline can bring on fright or apprehension. Heavy doses of noradrenaline increase fighting behavior in cats and mice; lowering the level of the chemical in the brain calms the animals. However, deficiency of noradrenaline at brain cell junctions in experimental animals has induced severe depression.

Some hormones at brain cell junctions are chemically related to some of the psychoactive drugs. Recently, a group of investigators (Cox *et al.*, 1975) isolated from the pituitary of cows and pigs what appears to be a new hormonal substance, POP-1 (pituitary opioid peptide 1). The effect of this substance on animal tissue is similar to that of opiates, and the researchers speculate that it will also have an opiatelike effect on mood. An intriguing aspect of the new discovery is that, although part of POP-1 molecule is like other pituitary hormone molecules (it is a peptide), POP-1 also contains a chemical residue similar to that of an opiate. Thus opiates may actually resemble the active chemical group in one of the pituitary hormones, POP-1, and the action of opiates may be the mimicking of some of the action of this hormone.

Even a stimulant as mild as coffee affects someone sensitive to caffeine, producing a mood change and inducing the jitters. Stimulants and depressants are more powerful, mood-changing sensual drugs. Some so-called mood-altering drugs such as marijuana and most hallucinogens, however, do not reverse a user's mood, but rather intensify the mood the user was already in. This can make a user believe he has actually altered his mood, but he usually discovers that the change is one of degree, not of quality. However, the more powerful drugs, opiates in particular, may completely eliminate unpleasant thoughts for a time and in this way alter a depressed mood to one of relief and happiness.

Stimulation of the pleasure centers

Some drugs seem to stimulate the pleasure centers directly – like drug or electrode stimulation of the limbic area in experimental animals and human subjects. This is probably true of the depressants and stimulants. Other drugs seem to stimulate the pleasure centers indirectly, distorting sensory information, memory, and thought. When pleasure is experienced from these drugs, it is usually *learned* pleasure. That is, the conscious brain must learn through conditioning that certain distortions of the senses are pleasurable. This is particularly true of the hallucinogenic drugs. The first time an individual loses his balance, forgets what he has just done, loses control of some muscles, or sees things that do not exist, it may be a frightening experience. However, he may learn to enjoy the bizarre, unexpected effects of the drug. In other words, the brain interprets the raw sensory data it receives. Depending on past experiences and on the present mental and physical state of the user, the drug experience can be interpreted as pleasurable or horrifying. Even the sensations from such a

mild hallucinogen as marijuana must be learned to be interpreted as pleasurable.

Pleasurable sensations

A drug can penetrate any number and combination of the
brain's capillaries to influence brain cells and produce a
variety of simultaneous sensations. As we have seen, the
limbic region alone controls many pleasurable sensations
and emotions, and there may be other pleasure areas outside the limbic region. Sensations are also determined by
such variables as dose, individual differences, environment,
immediate circumstances, and expectations. Thus, not
only do the sensations from any one drug vary, but not all
people can interpret the sensations as pleasurable.

To list the pleasurable effects for each of the drugs would
be lengthy and often repetitive, so I shall present some of
the characteristic sensations and moods most often described to me by drug users.

Well-being. This sensation is the one most often described
by drug users. In the healthy individual, each of the senses
contributes in its own way to the general feeling of well-
being. The feeling simply indicates that all the systems and
controls are functioning properly. Sensual drugs provide
this sensation by bypassing the senses and systems that report to the brain "all is well." They essentially fool the brain
into believing that all is operating normally. In a conditioned drug user, the brain's mechanisms become adjusted to the drug, with the result that the user feels well
only when the drug is present in the brain. All the sensual
drugs impart an artificial sense of well-being, and as dependency on these drugs becomes a way of life, the user depends for his sense of well-being on drugs and cannot respond to the natural sensations.

Euphoria. Euphoria is an intense feeling of well-being, often caused by an outpouring of adrenaline or the taking of stimulant drugs. Euphoria can also be induced by an excess of steroid hormones, especially the adrenal hormone, cortisone. Euphoria induced by steroid hormones lasts longer than that initiated by stimulants or adrenaline. Probably these chemical substances, whether hormones or drugs, imitate the feelings of euphoria directly in the brain's pleasure centers, for this effect seems to be felt no matter what the circumstances.

Sex. Many people report that certain drugs produce the same excitement or satiating, orgasmic relief that sexual activity does. Apparently that part of the limbic region in the brain where nerve tracts from erotic areas connect with the autonomic nervous system's controls for the sexual functions is stimulated. In other words, the sexlike sensations from drugs are produced in the brain and not through the normal mechanisms of the sex organs.

Loss of inhibition. The intoxicants (alcohol, barbiturates, tranquilizers, volatile solvents, and marijuana) cause a lowering of inhibitions. In the case of marijuana, this can persist long after the period of acute intoxication. The lowering of inhibitions seems proportional to the degree of intoxication. Apparently, controlling powers of the frontal lobes of the cerebral cortex (the conscious brain) are partially blocked or their function is diminished, so that impulses to act, generated in the lower parts of the brain, are not held in check. Some observers have characterized this as a carefree attitude and appearance. Certainly marijuana users seem often to be induced to participate in activities they would normally not consider.

Alertness. The stimulant drugs are often used in small doses to increase wakefulness and alertness and to extend the duration of physical activity that is dependent on alertness. Stimulants simultaneously increase the control of the sympathetic nervous system and correspondingly decrease the dominance of the parasympathetic nervous system; they increase heartbeat, blood pressure, and temperature, and release extra adrenaline into the system. Although the user feels clear-headed, this is not his true condition. The stimulants also cause hallucinations and errors in deduction. In large enough doses, they produce sensations of excitement and pleasure, but also, in some cases, agitation and delirium that can lead to impetuous behavior.

Relaxation. The minor depressant drugs (tranquilizers and sedatives) can be used to calm hyperactive or nervous people, to reduce tension, and to bring on sleep. They accomplish this by slowing the rate of internal functions and adrenaline production or by limiting the amount of sensory data that reaches the brain. The depressant drugs increase the relative control of the parasympathetic nervous system and decrease the dominance of the sympathetic system, thus lowering blood pressure, heartbeat, temperature, and adrenaline production.

Dizziness. Dizziness or light-headedness is associated with the use of intoxicants and seems to be the result of failure in the correlative control centers for balance and equilibrium. Similar disturbances result from impairment of the organs of equilibrium in the inner ear. Drugs that induce dizziness probably do not affect the organs of equilibrium, but rather the various centers that correlate sensations of position, motion, and acceleration. The sensation of dizziness is often concurrent with a distortion of visual correlative control centers that focus and stabilize objects. This makes the world seen to swim. Atropine (belladonna) and chemically related drugs, used to prevent seasickness, can depress the mental sensations of dizziness but may actually increase dizziness when used with an intoxicant.

Time distortion. Most of the sensual drugs interfere with short-term memory and distort other sensory perceptions. The scrambling affects the mind's ability to perceive lapses in time and the sequence of events and impairs the attention span and the power of concentration. Marijuana, especially, makes the user overestimate time. "Felt" time becomes longer than clock time. Alcohol, on the other hand, causes the user to underestimate the duration of time: he thinks it has passed faster than it actually has. One explanation is that the sense of time depends on the memory's evaluation of the number of sensory impressions received, which the hallucinogens increase and the intoxicants decrease.

Illusions. Illusions are unreal or misleading images and false ideas and interpretations originating within the brain. All the sensual drugs can produce illusions. The illusions produced by the hallucinogenic drugs are particularly intense. They cause a scrambling of the memory and distortion of sensory information to create an entirely different "reality." Often there is a telescoping of past, present, and future. Not only is the sensory world distorted, but the user may lead his life under a set of false notions about himself and others. The novelty of the experience may be fascinating, but it can easily turn into a terrifying bad trip.

CHAPTER 4

Hazards of sensual drugs

If drugs offered a safe form of pleasure, there might be few objections to using them. However, the claims that they are safe must be recognized as false in the face of the known consequences of continued drug use. Real dangers exist, although the drug user often assumes they do not because the harmful side effects are not immediately apparent. Possible results range from incidental deleterious effects to death from overdose; the dangers that lie between the extremes are the degeneration of health and the depletion of brain function. Drugs, after all, act directly on the brain and cause mental mechanisms to respond abnormally. The risks are great for the persistent user. In particular, there is danger that he will do himself a great deal of harm before the warning symptoms occur.

Drug-related health disorders are many and varied. Dirty needles and solutions used for injecting drugs can cause abscesses in the arms and veins, liver disease, venereal disease, and infections of the kidneys and brain. Sniffing cocaine and amphetamines can damage the tissue of the nose, and marijuana and tobacco smoking can cause lung disease. Heavy users of alcohol, volatile solvents, amphetamines, or marijuana may find that their livers are permanently damaged. Babies of women addicted to opiates are likely to be born addicted and to suffer from withdrawal symptoms. Cocaine and amphetamines can cause hair to fall out. Recent research has indicated that marijuana can damage cells. A drug user's way of life makes him more susceptible to pneumonia, tuberculosis, malnutrition, and weight loss. Finally, an overdose of any of the sensual drugs can lead to respiratory or cardiac failure and death.

This book focuses on the effects of drugs on the brain. This is not to minimize their effects on other parts of the body, for these can sometimes be more debilitating. Damage to the brain, however, is the most subtle, most often unrecognized, and least understood consequence of drug abuse.

Brain cell damage

Sensual drugs affect the chemistry of the brain cells. Cell function is carried out by thousands of enzymes acting within each cell. Depending on how the cell chemistry adds up, the cell either reinforces or shifts the dominance of cell pathways and hookups. Each exposure of the cells to psychoactive drugs somehow alters their chemistry. Most studies agree that cells can recover from exposure to a low dose, but in certain instances, high doses and chronic use have been toxic. Toxic effects may be transitory or permanent, depending on the nature of the cell damage.

The brain is composed mainly of brain nerve cells (*neurons*), blood vessels, supportive cells (*glia*), and insulating fat. The estimated 10 billion (American billion; 10,000,000,000) nerve cells form the substance of the brain through which thinking and feeling are carried on and by which brain messages are sent and received. Each nerve cell has three parts: a cell body, one fingerlike fiber (*axon*), and many spreading extensions of the cell body (*dendrites*) that carry (or inhibit) the nerve impulses to and from other nerve cells. The dendrites of each brain nerve cell branch out to make about 5,000 connections with other brain nerve cells; some are thought to make as many as 60,000 connections. The brain is estimated to have 50 trillion such *synaptic junctions* (junctions between cells). Messages are carried across or inhibited at these junctions by electrochemical controls. Thus, nerve cells communicate through waves of chemical changes sent along nerve pathways. Toxic chemicals can easily upset the delicate chemical balance of the brain's intricate system of communication; they may also damage cell tissue.

Laboratory methods for detecting brain cell damage

Drugs cause chemical damage to brain cells either by direct action or indirectly through anoxia (lack of oxygen). The damage may be cell death, cell injury, or disturbances at the synaptic junctions between cells. Damage to brain cells can be determined by x-ray examination, measurement of brain weight changes, analysis of brain wave changes, and microscopic examination of a sample of brain tissue. X-rays can detect only the massive cell loss that sometimes occurs in alcoholism and senility, when the brain shrinks away from the skull. Measurement of the weight change of brain tissue is a method used in animal studies to detect brain damage. The brains of experimental and control animals are weighed. A significant decrease in brain weight of the experimental animals indicates atrophy; an increase may be due to edema.

The waves of chemical change along the communicating nerve pathways cause a shift of ions, which results in a measurable electrical charge. Certain types of brain damage can be detected by altered electrical patterns of neuron action, measured by EEG (electroencephalography). EEG measures the average electrical charge at any one moment in certain areas of the brain. These are graphically recorded as brain waves. EEG provides a gross reflection of the electrical activity going on at the same time in various areas of the brain. Brain wave patterns are different from person to person, but after becoming established in the late teen years, the patterns remain remarkably consistent in each individual.

When electrodes are placed on the surface of the scalp, they record neuron activity in areas of the cerebral cortex (external layer of the brain). The patterns vary with mental activity and mood, and can sometimes be used to diagnose certain malfunctions such as epilepsy, tumors, physical injury, and episodic psychomotor disturbances.

The usefulness of brain waves as an indication of brain function increases as specific portions of the brain are monitored. New specialized devices can monitor electrical charges deep within the brain, but the procedure is delicate and risky. Electrodes are placed deep in the brain, adjacent to the many specialized centers of brain reflex activity. The electrical activity recorded may be linked to discrete sensory or motor activities not detectable in externally monitored brain waves. Although EEG can indicate brain damage, it cannot be used to determine whether the change in electrical charge is due to injured neurons, destroyed neurons, disturbance at the synapse, or a combination of these.

Microscopic examination of samples of brain tissue can directly detect brain cell loss. Tissue sections must be prepared immediately after death because the brain cells die within a few minutes after the blood supply is interrupted. A count of the brain nerve cells visible in the microscopic field indicates whether the brain has atrophied.

Brain cells are compactly assembled and complex in their interconnections – much more so than other body cells. Brain cells are so small that it has been estimated that 1 million could fit on the head of a pin. The loss of brain cells must be considerable, then, to establish that there are fewer nerve cells than expected in a particular specimen.

The fine neuron membranes and the interneuron connections are probably the most affected by toxic substances. The ordinary light microscope is unable to show enough about such structural details. Scanning and transmission electron microscopes are very new tools. They can magnify up to 100,000 times (compared with 900 times for an ordinary light microscope). The scanning electron microscope permits a comprehensive viewing of the surface structures, while the transmission electron microscope permits viewing of the interior of cells. Brain cells have been photographed with the use of these microscopes (Nilsson and Hydén, 1971). These electron microscopes have just begun to be used for brain cell research. They are currently used to view the synapse in the study of the effects of drug abuse on the delicate functional structures of the brain cells.

Difficulty in identifying brain cell damage

Drug users demand proof that a drug damages brain cells before they consider the drug harmful. What they fail to understand, however, is how difficult it is to identify brain cell damage, either in humans or in experimental animals – even when specimens are taken under the most favorable conditions. The brain is highly complex and compact, with folds, creases, billions of nerve cells, and thousands of nerve pathways. When damage is massive and localized, from a blow on the head or a tumor, for instance, damaged areas can be identified under the microscope. When the sensory and motor pathways are well understood and defined, the cause for the interruption of certain body functions can possibly be located in the brain at a postmortem examination because the investigator knows what he is looking for.

Thought pathways, on the other hand, are not well defined, and it is impossible, using present methods of microscopic examination, to inspect damage to cells affecting thought formation. When the damage is subtle and diffuse, as it is from certain toxic substances, locating such damage is at present almost impossible. When the "thinking" cells are damaged, a matrix of supporting cells remains, giving the brain a normal appearance. Although the quality of the thinking may be affected, the brain still functions to some extent from the reserves that are left.

It must not be assumed that because damaged brain cells cannot be identified under the microscope that none exist. For example, although opiate users often appear to recover from the effects of low-dose use, brain cell damage from high doses of opiates has been detected at postmortem examination; and it would seem likely that the disrupted thought patterns induced by smaller doses are an indication that some harm has been done – even though the damage cannot be detected under the microscope.

Certain cause-and-effect relationships have been discovered between brain malfunction and brain cell damage. When certain symptoms are evident, the researcher knows where to look for the brain cell damage. For example, it is now well established that the most prominent symptoms of senility are accompanied by marked deletions of brain cells. It took many years to establish this fact because the brains of the senile look quite normal on gross or microscopic examinations. Special techniques and painstaking work were necessary to show the thinning of the cells.

Brain cell damage from toxic chemicals

Microscopic examinations of brain cells from individuals who died of drug overdose and from experimental animals that were given large drug doses show that extensive structural changes have taken place. Under an ordinary light microscope, brain cells sickened by toxins show such nonspecific changes as swelling, lack of pigment granules, resistance to histological stain, and accumulation of clear fluid or fat droplets. Lighter staining of cells implies that the metabolic systems in the cells that convert food into energy are affected. In some cases, rather than metabolizing, the fat accumulates as droplets within the cells.

Such damage cannot be satisfactorily measured by x-ray examination or weight loss determination. This is because the smaller supportive cells and structures remain even though some neurons have disappeared. For example, in brains damaged by solvent poisoning (such as from solvents of plastic glue, ether, benzene, or alcohol) or senility, microscopic examination shows the dense supportive structures intact and a thinning of the neurons. This is not strikingly evident on x-ray examination or weight loss determination because the pockets containing the absent neurons remain, giving the impression that the cells are still there.

The progressive disappearance of brain cells owing to chronic exposure to toxic substances is comparable to an acceleration of the process of aging. The first step in the process is the sickening of brain cells, with the accompanying changes mentioned above.

Since THC (tetrahydrocannabinol, the active ingredient in marijuana) was isolated, many studies have been done on its effect on the brain. Alteration of cell membranes and functions and shrinkage of midbrain structures have been noted. Given doses corresponding to those used by humans, experimental monkeys showed significant organic brain damage. Brain wave changes have been noted in cases of marijuana-induced psychosis. (Brain damage from marijuana use is discussed more fully in Chapter 10.)

Anoxia, caused most often by the intoxicants and stimu-

lants, can damage brain cells. The cells are critically dependent on a steady supply of oxygen from the blood. The
brain has a protective system: when its oxygen supply is
failing, the capillaries expand to receive more blood. However, when the capillaries expand to their maximum size,
they occasionally burst or leak blood, causing a tiny hemorrhage around each broken vessel. This further reduces the
supply of blood and oxygen to that area.

Intoxicants often interfere with the entry of oxygen and
the utilization of oxygen in the cells. The brain's powerful
mechanisms try to compensate for this anoxia, but the increased blood flow is sometimes insufficient, and cell damage results. High doses of drugs that prevent oxygen from
reaching brain cells often lead to hemorrhage and greater
cell destruction.

Stimulants may affect the oxygen level in brain cells
either directly, by constricting small arteries and capillaries,
or indirectly, by causing a massive release of adrenaline. In
either case, small arteries of the brain constrict, sometimes
enough to stop the flow of blood. After the stimulant has
worn off, the regions deprived of oxygen may hemorrhage.
Multiple hemorrhages in the brain tissue are usually found
in victims of a fatal dose of stimulants. People I have interviewed who have taken massive doses of amphetamines or
cocaine suffer from what Widroe (1975) has called "grossly
scattered thinking," impaired speech, and residual tremor.
These are usually the symptoms of the random, multiple
hemorrhaging in the brain of an older person who has had a
series of small strokes. The condition does not pass quickly.
Former amphetamine addicts show symptoms of "cortical
impairment" months after they have stopped taking drugs.

In cases of severe poisoning by amanita mushrooms,
brain cell damage and small hemorrhages have been found.
Because mescaline, psilocybin, and LSD have active ingredients similar to those in amanita mushrooms and have

similar hallucinogenic effects, it is possible that they have a similar effect on brain cells. These powerful hallucinogens must also dislocate some reflex nerve pathways. In experiments on spiders under the influence of LSD, this effect has been clearly demonstrated. The spiders consistently leave out portions of their usual web pattern, indicating that there has been permanent damage to their nervous systems. Some spiders have permanent impairment after a single dose of LSD (Groh & Lemieux, 1968).

Although high doses of drugs do the greatest damage to brain cells, there are indications that the cumulative effect of lower doses may be injurious as well. Chronic alcoholism is an example. In several marginal brain diseases, even a slight exposure to drugs may cause functional difficulty, indicating that the effects of the disease and the drug are additive, for example, an anesthetic may be hazardous to a person suffering with brain syphilis or may precipitate an attack in a person having multiple sclerosis. Alcoholics, though more resistant to anesthesia, may develop more complications in their brain cells from the use of anesthetics than the normal person would. These observations indicate that weakened brain cells cannot tolerate as much chemical interference as healthy cells can.

Although dead brain cells cannot regenerate, swollen and sick brain cells can recover, up to a point. Chemical mechanisms at the synapses that normally transmit impulses between cells adjust themselves to respond to a toxic chemical disturbance. In addition, it has been established that neurons can develop new axonal or dendritic connections:

Cut axons have been found to sprout vigorously new axons that enter and supply nerves to structures in the brain not previously innervated by this group of axons. In areas where innervation has been removed, the monoamine producing axons appear to sprout and re-innervate the vacated synaptic sites. A related observation is that nerve cells near damaged cells move in to fill the vacancy. This filling in process may be interpreted as a form of reorganization. [Widroe, 1975]

Widroe refers to the development of these new connections as "re-wiring." He has conjectured that this process is responsible for the effective training of brain-damaged patients.

Brain cells obviously must survive even after structural and functional disturbances. Otherwise, alcoholics, for example, would soon be depleted of irreplaceable brain cells. Loss of functional capacity and a shortened life span of the brain cells are, however, known risks of drug abuse. Atrophy of the brain (loss of brain cells) occurs earlier and is more severe in individuals who have been consistently exposed to toxic substances.

Some effects of drugs on brain cells can only be deduced from what are known to be the symptoms of brain damage. When a young drug user shows signs of senility, it can be deduced that he has lost some brain cell function. In contrast to the truly senile person, however, some of the damaged cells of the drug user may recover after a period of abstinence. Whether all recover is an unanswered question. The chronic user of alcohol, barbiturates, tranquilizers, amphetamines, marijuana, or cocaine may develop symptoms of Parkinson's disease, a disorder associated with aging and caused by brain atrophy. He develops a masklike expression and a tremor; the loss of other mental powers may follow in later stages. Tremor is a common complication of drug use. It may appear at first only when the drug is withdrawn. This typically happens to those dependent on coffee or alcohol. With longer exposure and more extensive brain changes, tremor is likely to be persistent.

A drug user may suffer bewilderment or memory difficulties during a drug-free interval. This may indicate transient or permanent brain damage. Some individuals who become neurotic or psychotic through drug abuse or bad trips may be described as psychically disturbed. However, it is necessary to explain the psychic illness in functional terms. Certainly, in some cases of drug-induced psychic illness, changes in brain wave patterns are an indication of physical impairment. They are probably caused by some persistent, functional impairment. Also, when the drug user is unable to recover from the drug's effects on his brain, especially after a long period of abstinence, it must be assumed that there has been some form of permanent damage to the brain cells.

It has increasingly become recognized that some mental disturbances are related to the chemistry of the brain nerve cells. In fact, drugs are now being prescribed to treat certain forms of mental illness. It seems that drugs can both balance and unbalance brain cell chemistry.

Sensory deprivation

This tragic aspect of drug abuse is usually left undiscussed. Sensory deprivation occurs with the use of all the sensual drugs, but most notably with the use of the opiates. The drug user reaches a state where his ability to relate to sensations is diminished because of drug use. A kind of paranoia is produced. The senses – touch, hearing, or vision – are suppressed, and the subject becomes ill at ease and uncomfortable.

The addict loses his capacity to enjoy even the simplest pleasures of life. He may suffer from impotence, and his sexual development may be disrupted. Because drugs induce feelings of pleasure directly in the brain, the pleasure they bring gradually supplants the normal stimulations of thought and the senses. As a result, the brain eventually becomes conditioned to respond only to the drug's stimulation. This is both a psychological and a physical phenomenon. At first, the pleasurable sensations are enhanced as the controls are artificially stimulated; then, the normal pathways in the brain become progressively less responsive. Finally, they may fail altogether, so that even the drug cannot stimulate them.

During the buildup of tolerance to a drug, the ability of the natural sensations to stimulate pleasure diminishes. With prolonged drug use, fewer and fewer sensations or thoughts stimulate the pleasure centers, and the drug user comes to be virtually without emotion. Only the drug gives pleasure, and even that pleasure fades as the controls adjust and become tolerant to the drug. The variety and distinction of feelings are reduced, and the only clear desire is for the drug. This desire, which is at first the desire for pleasure, eventually becomes the desire to avoid the misery of withdrawal. Thus, in bypassing the safeguards that protect the pleasure mechanism, the drug eventually causes failure in the very mechanism that produced the pleasurable sensations.

The depth of the emotional depression felt by some heroin addicts was revealed to me when I interviewed them. After they had become addicted, they were unable to appreciate most of the things that once gave them pleasure: friends, family, sexual stimulation, physical comfort, food, and sleep. The GI heroin addicts I interviewed in Vietnam had stopped writing letters home. They had stopped writing, they said, not because they didn't want to correspond, not because they were too preoccupied with their drug experiences to do so, but because they felt too disconnected from those at home to bother.

These multiple emotional changes in the drug user are a consequence of sensory deprivation. Continued drug use causes the abnormal patterns of response to become the usual ones, and the alterations of personality and outlook become permanent. The opiate addict severs himself from those who care about him and thus reinforces his sense of isolation and loneliness. He is troubled by the lack of warm response from companions and imagines that they dislike or hate him. Indifference, depression, and hustling to get drugs are soon the limits of his dealings with the world, and he is left without the channels that normally would help him maintain emotional maturity and health.

The opiate user also experiences the loss of sexual capacity. Not only is the ability to feel sexual sensations suppressed, but the desire for sex is lost as well. The addict is able to retain the overwhelming pleasure of the opiate only because he increases the dose. When his senses fully tolerate the highest doses – when, as the addicts say, he is burned out – he is as unresponsive to opiates as he is to sex. No sensations can give him pleasure. An addict may undergo withdrawal so he can renew his sensitivity to opiates, but this does not fully restore his emotional or sexual powers. By the age of thirty-five, an addict may be totally unresponsive both to drugs and to normal emotions.

Lesser forms of sensory deprivation can be seen in chronic users of other drugs. Over a relatively short time, the chronic smoker finds his senses of taste and smell and his ability to enjoy tobacco are diminished. In users of both alcohol and marijuana, sensations from the body diminish as drug use continues. The early effects seem to be reversible. The senses are regained after a period of abstinence, but if chronic, heavy use has gone on too long, abstinence can bring little or no recovery.

Impaired memory and reason

When the sensual drugs distort sensory information and disrupt memory, the false information produced disturbs the reasoning faculties. Sensory information is disturbed by the drug's effects on correlative control centers. Thus, even if the drug does not actually affect the cells of the cerebral cortex appreciably, the reasoning faculties must try to deal with distorted information and cannot operate efficiently.

As illusionary experiences increase, it becomes difficult for the brain to sort out what is real from what is not. Reasoning and thought formation become confused, and responses, based on distortions, are often unrealistic and inappropriate.

Reasoning is made even more difficult when a drug affects the memory storage facility. Goals cannot be kept in mind and thoughts wander. Thoughts and events cannot be held in the brain for any length of time, so cause-and-effect relationships and logical progessions cannot be perceived. Even the simplest decisions, such as, Shall I sit down? are difficult to make. When sensory information and memory retention are impaired, even this sort of question can be perplexing, and very often it cannot be differentiated from other, more important questions.

If the senses are severely distorted, as they can be by hallucinogens, the reasoning faculties have no basis on which to work and act. The records contain many reports of drug users who, while hallucinating, think they can fly or see people who are not there, who hear unreal voices, or who dissociate completely from their bodies. They become depersonalized. When distorted sensory information is passed on to the higher portions of the brain, it is virtually impossible to act rationally. When such information gets implanted in long-term memory, irrational behavior can be permanent.

The last effect is apparent in flashbacks. Evidently, the original experience is firmly implanted in the memory and can occur again in the mind without warning or at the merest suggestion of the original experience.

Because the natural means of stimulating the control centers are bypassed, a drug can produce a sense of well-being even when the information the body receives should indicate otherwise. The drug forces the brain to interpret the true state of the body falsely. The individual may have no sensation of pain although his body may actually be damaged. He may have sensations of euphoria while surrounded by tragedy; he may feel well when he is actually sick; or he may feel wide awake when his body needs rest. The body and brain become susceptible to physical damage and harmful suggestions as information the brain needs for its survival becomes confused. A false sense of security and indestructibility predominates. Reason becomes unreliable, and the drug user is unable to make decisions and direct himself away from dangerous situations.

Alteration of the diurnal cycle

Drugs used in sufficient doses can distort the concept of time. As dependency increases, the drug user begins to stay awake at night and sleep during the day. The natural diurnal cycle is reversed. This change is often accompanied by an increased sensitivity of the eyes to light and a reduced awareness of the passage of time, such as seasons. Alteration of the diurnal cycle is pronounced with the use of marijuana, amphetamines, or narcotics.

Uncontrollable mood changes, psychotic reactions

Undesirable and uncontrollable changes in mood are one of the hazardous brain effects of sensual drug use. This is particularly noticeable during withdrawal, when the controls are in a state of readjustment and moods opposite to that produced by the drug are experienced. For example, drug-induced euphoria or exhilaration gives way to depression, or calmness is replaced by agitation, restlessness, and sleeplessness. These unpleasant changes in mood often provoke the user to take another dose. The alternate use of uppers and downers is often an attempt to control or redirect swings in moods. The drug user whose diurnal cycle is disturbed is likely to use chemicals to help him to maintain a schedule corresponding to the light/dark cycle. Drugs can cause abrupt changes in mood, such as the bursts of laughter or tears of the barbiturate user or the manic, high-strung restlessness of the cocaine or amphetamine user. Sometimes mood swings abruptly to flashes of unwarranted hostility, unprovoked rage, or violence. This occurs particularly with the use of large doses of amphetamines, cocaine, barbiturates, tranquilizers, or alcohol.

Drugs can disturb brain controls for memory, reasoning, and moods to such an extent that they cause varying degrees of psychotic reactions. The amphetamine psychosis of a speed freak, for example, is literally indistinguishable from paranoid schizophrenia. A Swedish psychiatrist (Bejerot, 1970*a*) who studied amphetamine users in Sweden described the symptoms of amphetamine psychosis as pronounced delusions of persecution, hallucinations of hearing, and intense anxiety, which may rise to violent terror. Although perhaps not as common, hallucinations of sight have also been reported. Amphetamine psychoses may persist for many years after the period of abuse (Tatetsu, as reviewed in Lemere, 1966). Cocaine can cause a similar psychosis. Dose, method of administration, length of time used, the experiences of the user, and genetic predisposition determine the severity of the cocaine psychosis (Post, 1975). An LSD user can undergo a personality change much like that of a simple schizophrenic: " [the user] becomes vague, somewhat confused, and dependent on the group for his own fading personality identity. His sense of purpose and his will grow pale, like a color picture long exposed to sunlight" (R. Campbell, 1971).

Over a century ago, Moreau found hashish users had symptoms similar to those of the mentally ill. Moreau and his pupils took many different size doses of hashish and made detailed notes during their intoxications. They observed each other carefully and discussed their impressions, feelings, and thoughts before, during, and after the experience. In 1845, as a result of his systematic experimentation, Moreau published a book, *Du hachich et de l'alienation mentale: études psychologiques*. (Alienation was then the common term used to describe mental illness.) In it he stated: "I have compared the principal characteristics observed in mental illness to the symptoms caused in me by hashish intoxication. The insights provided by my own study gave me a better understanding of mental illness" (Moreau, 1845).

One of the effects of many of the sensual drugs is a disorganization of the sense of time. This is also a prominent symptom of paranoid delusion, and temporal disorganization has been associated with schizophrenic thought disorders (Bleuler, 1950). In experiments, high doses of THC have been used to induce a disorganized sense of time in carefully screened, normal subjects (Melges *et al.*, 1974). It was found that in all subjects, there were substantial changes linking temporal disorganization and delusional thoughts. The researchers concluded that "temporal disorganization and delusional-like ideation are mutually interacting processes."

Change of life style

Heavy drug use causes changes in life style. Some commonly noted consequences of heavy drug use are decreased motivation, less goal orientation, a loss of inhibitions, and susceptibility to suggestion. The changes may vary according to the type and amount of drug used and to individual differences. The young drug user's brain seems particularly vulnerable. In general, the changes appear slowly with the abuse of alcohol, gradually and cumulatively with marijuana, and strikingly with heroin, barbiturates, tranquilizers, cocaine, and amphetamines. Cocaine and amphetamine users may be motivated toward unrealistic goals and be unable to perceive the real situation.

Sometimes the changes are explained as the result of shifts in environment – a change in friends from non users to drug users. This is no doubt a factor; but what people do not take seriously enough is the possibility (and in my opinion the probability) that the user's whole outlook – not just cognitive function or mood – is altered by the heavy use of sensual drugs. The amotivational syndrome of the heavy user of marijuana is a good illustration. This syndrome is now considered by authorities to be a direct effect of the drug on the brain. Case histories have documented (Kolansky & Moore, 1972b) that the personality changes of marijuana users occur subsequent to marijuana smoking and not as the result of social changes. I have observed changes of life style in many young people who were well known to me before they used marijuana; I have also seen them become motivated and goal-oriented again when they stopped using marijuana. The impairment of the thinking process, particularly the ability to distinguish the sequence of events, may in some way play a part in the decline in goal orientation of drug users.

One physician related to me how she became addicted to amphetamines. She used them regularly as a medical student to counteract fatigue and drowsiness. She progressed to heavy, compulsive abuse. She dropped out of medical school and completely changed her way of life. Among other distinct changes, she became preoccupied with sex. Ultimately she went through rehabilitation twice, at great expense, after being persuaded by her family. She eventually recovered from the effects of her long addiction and completed her medical studies. Many case histories of people who have changed their life style after drug use are recorded. Some are written by rehabilitated addicts; some by parents of addicts. *Wasted: The Story of My Son's Drug Addiction*, by William Chapin, is one such account.

Overdose

The greatest danger in the use of the depressant and intoxicant drugs is that there is such a fine line between sensual and poisonous effects: a toxic dose is only a few times greater than that used for medical purposes. As the dose is raised to maintain pleasurable effects, the drug may more severely affect the controls for the vital organs, since both the pleasure centers and the autonomic controls are located in the limbic region. Thus, the pleasure centers react to large doses of the opiates, barbiturates, tranquilizers, volatile solvents, and alcohol, but breathing, heart action, and blood pressure are, at the same time, depressed. The results can be dizziness, confusion, convulsions, unconsciousness, or death. Appendix 1 gives estimates of the amounts of some of the commonly used psychoactive drugs that can cause intoxication or unconsciousness. It is particularly hazardous to take depressant and intoxicant drugs in combination because sublethal doses of individual drugs may become lethal when combined. In fact, the user can never be completely sure of his reaction to any combination of the sensual drugs.

Alcohol, barbiturates, and tranquilizers are sometimes taken by opiate or amphetamine users. Amphetamine users take barbiturates or tranquilizers to bring themselves down to a more restful mental state or to mitigate the effects of withdrawal. Those who have become dependent on the sexual rush that accompanies opiate injection sometimes inject themselves with alcohol, barbiturates, or tranquilizers when heroin is not available. This is as dangerous as injecting the opiate: some unmixed, undiluted portions of the injected barbiturate or tranquilizer may find their way to the vital control centers and produce instant heart or respiratory failure. Within the drug culture, death from overdose of barbiturates taken either orally or by injection is nearly as common as death from herion or methodone overdose. Deaths from overdose of tranquilizers have also occurred. The tranquilizer diazepam (Valium) has become one of the more commonly abused drugs in Massachusetts, a fact that is apparent from the number of users applying to the emergency wards of the city's hospitals (Patch, 1974).

Amyl nitrite, a depressant, is used as an aphrodisiac just before sexual climax to augment orgasmic sensations. It produces a rapid decline in blood pressure that, together with the postorgasmic circulatory changes, can quickly cause circulatory collapse, heart arrest, unconsciousness, and death.

Large doses of stimulants or hallucinogens also can cause failure of the vital control centers, but because these drugs stimulate rather than suppress vital functions, abuse is less likely to be fatal. Nevertheless, lethal overdose does sometimes occur. High doses of these drugs can produce unconsciousness because they can abruptly shift from stimulating nerves to stopping nerve action. Cocaine is such a stimulant. At high doses it can interfere with certain nerve actions – possibly because it is a powerful local anesthetic. Acute cocaine poisoning comes on rapidly, especially when the drug is injected. Difficulty with respiration usually precedes convulsions and unconsciousness. In some instances, the symptoms develop so rapidly that the acute intoxication results in almost immediate death.

Death from marijuana smoking is very rare. However, what part marijuana smoking plays in intensifying the toxic effects of other drugs used in combination with it is difficult to determine. Two deaths have been attributed to oral overdoses of marijuana (Ames, 1958), and several instances of highly toxic reactions to intravenous use of marijuana have been reported (Payne & Brand, 1975). There are many observations in the older literature of the oral therapeutic application of cannabis resin or its tincture under medical supervision causing convulsions, disturbances of the central nervous system, partial paralysis, and cardiac and respiratory distress.

CHAPTER 5

Addiction and dependency

Precisely how an individual will react to a drug is not easy to predict because his body chemistry, the circumstances, and the nature of the drug are all variables. Usually, drug experiments do not lead to compulsive or heavy use; yet some people become heavy users soon after the first experiment. Some drugs are simply more addictive than others, and some people are more susceptible to drugs than other people. Of every six people who use alcohol extensively, only one will become an alcoholic, and it will probably take him many years. At the other extreme, the daily use of opiates can develop into addiction within a few days.

I do not believe, as some do, that there is an addictive personality; but I do believe that certain individuals are more susceptible than others, to the compulsive use of drugs and that no person is immune to the risk of compulsive drug use. Anyone can become an addict with sufficient exposure. The key to compulsive drug use is that the individual finds a reason to like the experience. Sometimes a particularly responsive body chemistry is a factor in the response; sometimes social conditions are the reason for continued use. Most often, abuse is the result of a combination of psychological orientation and the social context within which the drug is offered.

74

What is drug addiction?

Many authorities, although they realize that certian drugs can create psychological dependencies, do not call a drug addictive unless there is also evidence of a chemical dependency – that is, unless there is an obvious buildup of tolerance with continued use and unless the abstinence syndrome appears when the drug is withdrawn. Drug use that appears to be motivated by a psychological craving is relegated to the category of mere habituation and thus is considered less harmful. I believe, however, that most sensual drugs are chemically addictive to some degree and can produce both tolerance and withdrawal symptoms.

Many people fail to recognize the close relationship between the two kinds of drug dependencies. Psychological and chemical addictions can be usefully separated for the purpose of discussion, but in reality they are two aspects of one problem. A person who regularly takes a drug for its sensual effects is dependent (or addicted) physically as well as psychologically. I maintain that there cannot be psychological addiction without at least some degree of chemical addiction. How the interactions between chemical and psychological functions of the brain work is unknown, but there is evidence that psychological changes affect the chemical balance of the body and that chemical alterations have psychological consequences. Even in 1926 the Rolleston Committee, whose recommendations set the policy for the treatment of narcotic addicts in England for forty-two years, recognized the link between psychological and physical dependency. They defined an addict as "a person who, not requiring the continued use of a drug for the relief of the symptoms of organic disease, has acquired, as a result of repeated administration, an overpowering desire for its continuance, and in whom withdrawal of the drug leads to definite symptoms of mental or physical distress or disorder"

(Great Britain, Ministry of Health, 1926). More recently, the World Health Organization in reference to sensual drugs rejected its earlier (1957) distinction between addiction and habituation on the grounds that the difference was purely semantic.

Because of the difficulty in trying to make a clear separation between the two dependencies, I will define *addiction* and *dependency* as any self-activating and compulsive tendency toward repetitive use of a drug. Thus, this book uses addiction and dependency interchangeably.

Becoming addicted

People start using the sensual drugs for many different psychological reasons: to relieve anxiety or depression, to escape the harshness of reality, for a thrill, or because of social pressures. The motivations are often unconscious and are highly individual. Understanding the compelling force of addiction is essential to the understanding of risk taking. For a young person to risk (often unknowingly) his sexual potency and to continue to take drugs even after his debilitation becomes obvious to him, the forces of psychological and chemical addiction must be very strong indeed.

Although addicts can often give a vivid picture of how and why they got hooked, it is difficult to reach below the surface of their words to discover the truth. Their stories are often inaccurate; addicts are notorious liars, and ex-addicts tend to rationalize rather than relate truthfully how they developed their dependencies. Studies of drug users, however, have revealed some basic patterns that seem to characterize the majority of the cases.

For the most part, the young drug user is not introduced to drugs by the fabled sly, seedy, corner pusher, but rather by a member of his own peer group who happens to have had more experience with drugs. The drug advocate is likely to be an older, more self-assured member of the group whose charisma inspires others to follow his example. Peer groups exert additional pressure on the novice. The urge to conform with a group to establish independence from adult authority is typical of the adolescent stage of emotional development, and the need for acceptance may cause the novice to succumb to peer pressure. The need for approval is not limited to the adolescent, however; it also motivates the older nonaddict to turn on and become hooked with an addict spouse or close friend.

The influence of friends on adolescents' drug use is shown in a study of over 8,000 New York high school students (Kandel, 1973). It was found that drug behavior in "best friends" was similar. In fact, in no other activity or attitude surveyed – school attitudes and performance, deviant behavior of various kinds, political attitudes, drug-related attitudes, and attitudes toward parents – was the similarity between friends as great as in their use of illegal drugs. For example, only 1 percent smoked marijuana sixty times or more if their friends had never smoked marijuana; 48 percent smoked marijuana if their friends had also smoked marijuana sixty times or more. A psychiatrist colleague who sees many marijuana users says he rarely finds a regular marijuana user who has not actively attempted to influence friends to try the drug (Powelson, personal communication).

The novice is dependent on the advocate at each step of the drug experience: for his first supply of the drug, for a demonstration of how to take it, and for information on what to expect from the first experience. The friend may offer some of his own supply; he may roll the first joint, count out the capsules, or even inject the drug into the vein of the novice.

The first time most people take drugs, the effects are unpleasant. This is especially true of tobacco, alcohol, and mescaline. With marijuana, the first-time effects are essentially nonexistent. If the user persists, it is usually because he is repeatedly urged on by the experienced friend who extolls the drug's more pleasurable features. After he has taken the drug several times, the novice finds that pleasurable sensations finally begin to overshadow the unpleasant effects, and he may find that the drug helps ease his social embarrassment.

Thus, drug use spreads from user to novice. A British investigator (de Alarcón, 1969) in interviews with heroin users found one person who had started using heroin in 1962. This user gave four other people their first fix. Two of these initiated others, and in five years time, thirty-two people had been initiated into heroin use through this chain. Another person who had started using heroin in 1965 initiated three others; in two years, sixteen users could be traced back along the chain to him. All these users were about the same age – between fifteen and twenty years old.

Many users become addicted to drugs after taking them to relieve pain. Morphine, amphetamines, and barbiturates are the drugs most commonly involved in this addiction syndrome (see below, under "Nonsensual use of drugs and addiction"). Sometimes a drug though not initially used for medical purposes, is found to have some medicinal properties and continues to be used for that reason. For example, some people have been known to continue to use marijuana for its analgesic (aspirinlike) action. Many marijuana smokers I have interviewed state that they find marijuana a good replacement for such drugs as aspirin, tranquilizers, or sedatives. In fact, it has been found that the electrical stimulation of an area for pleasure centers, the septal region of the brain, can relieve intractable physical pain. These connections between areas for pain and pleasure could offer a physiological basis for the analgesic effect of the sensual

drugs (Heath, 1972*a*). Relief from pain is, then, a strong
incentive to continue drug use.

Psychological conditioning

It is entirely normal for people to seek pleasure and avoid
pain. When a stimulus is found that produces pleasurable
sensations, it is equally normal for people to seek that
stimulus again and again. We tend to assume, however, that
if a certain effect is produced once or twice, it can be re-
created any number of times. We become accustomed to
associating a certain stimulus with pleasure. Before long,
even a suggestion of the stimulus can produce the response
associated with the pleasure. This is identical to the classical
Pavlovian conditioning: a bell is rung, food is presented,
and the dog salivates copiously; after a time, the dog salivates at the ringing of the bell alone.

The conditioning process cannot be considered the cause
of addiction, but it explains how an individual can unintentionally allow himself to become addicted. Not only does
his conscious mind become conditioned to pleasure-giving
stimuli, but as indicated by Pavlov's experiments, his autonomic reactions are also conditioned.

Conditioning for pleasure in humans begins in infancy.
The infant's life is governed by an instinctual drive to avoid
pain and achieve pleasure. He quickly learns to recognize
the cause-and-effect relationship between a specific pain
and the source of its relief. He learns to associate the uncomfortable fullness of his excretory tracts with the relief he
feels as he empties them; he associates fatigue with the restoration sleep brings; and hunger with the satisfaction of his
mother's milk.

The ways the infant learns to relieve pain and initiate
pleasure are reinforced by pleasure conditioning. Although
he will at first eat just about anything that is brought to him
to relieve his hunger, he soon develops preferences, espe-

cially for the familiar. After a certain point, his new preferences are not easily altered unless the change is associated with a compelling stimulus such as the approval of his parents or his peers. In this way, a child can be conditioned for or against any tastes, sights, smells, sounds, feelings, or activities by strong positive or negative associations. This is a form of behavioral conditioning.

Adult patterns of behavior are probably the result of both classical and behavioral conditioning. When sex, for example, becomes the dominant form of sensual gratification, it becomes its own powerful conditioning agent. Sensations and objects an individual associates with sex remain in his memory and subsequently influence his sexual behavior. Because he is likely to try to repeat the pleasurable experience, he finds that his sexual response mechanisms have become conditioned to that particular experience, just as the baby was conditioned to his favorite food. For instance, if he has been sexually aroused by a woman who wears a particular perfume, he may be aroused again whenever he smells that scent. This happens particularly if the initial encounter was pleasurable, frequently repeated, or especially memorable.

Occasionally, an individual is so strongly conditioned by the circumstances surrounding his sexual experiences that more and more of his attention is directed toward them rather than toward the sex act itself. When this happens, his desire for the provocative stimulation replaces his desire for natural sexual expression. This is a form of sexual deviation.

The compulsion to take drugs is also a form of pleasure conditioning. As the user continues to take a drug, he becomes accustomed to the physical pleasure and psychological satisfaction the drug gives him. Even though artificial, the stimulation of the pleasure mechanisms fulfills a profound psychological need for pleasure, and each successive titillation helps to reinforce the link between the drug and the emotional gratification. The persistent user begins to rely on and anticipate more and more the pleasurable sensations induced by the drug. He soon comes to feel a sense of emptiness that can be relieved only by taking the drug again. This sense of emptiness is due not so much to the absence of the newly discovered drug-induced sensations as to the fact that the pleasure mechanism has lost its ability to respond to natural stimulation. It is conditioned instead to expect the pleasure of the drug experience. Thus, the drug provides the impetus for a new pattern of behavior centered around the immediate gratification of the addict's sensual and psychological desires. Because this urge for satisfaction is strong, conditioning proceeds rapidly, and the new pattern soon takes precedence over almost all others.

This conditioning has one curious effect. Although tolerance gradually weakens the physiological impact of the drug, the addict continues, at least for some time, to get a sensual thrill. It appears that the diminishing effects of the drug are masked by a conditioned response. Just as Pavlov's dogs salivated at the ringing of the bell, the confirmed drug user can get some of the same effects from the mechanics of drug taking that he once could from the drug itself. For example, a junkie learns to expect the rush of sensual pleasure that follows an injection. Eventually, even injecting an inert substance gives him a kick and postpones withdrawal symptoms – as long as he thinks he is using heroin. The tobacco smoker develops a similar response. From the beginning, he learns to associate the effects of nicotine with watching the curls of smoke. Over years of heavy smoking, his response to the drug diminishes and he loses his sense of smell; but as long as he can watch the smoke, he enjoys his cigarette. Blindfolded, however, he cannot tell a lit from an unlit cigarette.

Early stages of chemical addiction

It is generally thought that prior to real addiction – that is, before withdrawal symptoms are experienced – a drug user can easily leave drugs alone. But my interviews with addict soldiers in Vietnam and drug users in the United States suggest that this is not entirely true. Before they become chemically addicted, most drug users do not feel well when they are without drugs, especially when they awaken in the morning. They take another dose to relieve the dreariness and to feel the drug's pleasurable impact. These initial symptoms are the forerunners of withdrawal symptoms. I found that they could result from a single use of heroin and could last for several weeks.

Such subtle, persistent changes in the body indicate a long-lasting, depressant effect on certain sensory correlative control functions. When drugs are withdrawn, even though withdrawal symptoms are not experienced, the body invites chemical intervention to restore its balance. If a drug user can be persuaded to stop at this early stage, he will not become addicted. If he continues, however, psychological and chemical dependencies will develop.

Chemical addiction

Chemical addiction occurs with the development of tolerance to a drug. Tolerance is a natural response of the chemical regulatory mechanisms to a substance that may have distressing or lethal effects. The various mechanisms adjust themselves so that they can function adequately in the presence of the drug and cannot perform properly without it.

Even though a drug directly influences only one group of control mechanisms, the effect soon spreads throughout the entire system. All the control centers, particularly those in the brain, compensate when one control center alters its function. As the centers readjust, the drug has less and less effect on physiological function, and the user must take bigger and bigger doses to attain a high. If the interval between doses is long enough to allow the controls to return to normal, chemical dependency is not established; the dose does not have to be increased to obtain the drug's effect.

However, when the control mechanisms have become so firmly reset that the drug is needed simply to maintain a functional balance, discontinuing its use results in a chemical and psychological imbalance that is manifested in the *abstinence syndrome*. The symptoms of this illness, the withdrawal symptoms, are the precise opposite of the symptoms of drug use. Heroin, for instance, produces a sense of well-being, constipation, and impotence and relieves itching or pain. Withdrawal results in psychological depression, diarrhea, a transitory return of disoriented sexual functions, and intense itching and pain. Withdrawal symptoms continue until the body readjusts to function normally without the drug. Although the major readjustments take place during detoxification, many important readjustments, such as the ability to sleep soundly, may not occur for months or even years.

Drug hunger

The craving the addict continues to have for a drug, long after he has been detoxified, is called *drug hunger*. It has been assumed that this is a psychological hunger; there are, however, indications that it may be the result of a long-lasting alteration of the brain's chemistry.

Reverse tolerance

Some of the sensual drugs can be taken in smaller and smaller doses and still produce the same effect; repeated doses of the same size produce increasingly greater effects. It has been argued that drugs showing these characteristics, usually marijuana, are not chemically addictive. Without a buildup of tolerance, it has been said, there can be no withdrawal symptoms.

The fact is that *reverse tolerance* occurs during only one stage of drug use; tolerance may still be built up during other stages. There are several causes of this build-up.

1. Changes may take place in organs outside the brain, especially the liver. For example, chronic heavy drinking damages the liver so it cannot remove as much alcohol from the blood as it could before it was damaged. The drinker then needs less alcohol to get the same sensual effects. He has, however, already built up a tolerance to large doses of alcohol before he reaches this stage. The person with a damaged liver also has a reverse tolerance for barbiturates, tranquilizers, and other drugs that are removed from the body through the liver.

2. The drug may accumulate in the body tissue. This occurs with marijuana. In the early periods of use, THC (tetrahydrocannabinol, the active principle in marijuana) accumulates in the body, and successive exposures to small doses cause increasingly sensual effects.

3. Brain cells may be irritated. With the chronic use of some drugs, notably cocaine, the sensitive brain cells become irritated so that smaller and smaller doses produce the sensual effect sought. Before this happens, however, there is usually a buildup of tolerance to large doses. This kind of sensitivity can be compared to the sensitivity of burned skin to hot water. Burned skin becomes sensitive even to warm water.

Individual drugs and chemical addiction

Tolerance and withdrawal symptoms are two criteria for determining if a drug is chemically addicting. Many factors influence the speed with which tolerance develops. Among them are how quickly the drug is absorbed or excreted and the susceptibility of the individual. In addition, each drug produces a variety of mental and physical effects, and tolerance does not necessarily develop to all of them at the same rate. Tolerance to some effects may not develop at all.

These points have been demonstrated in a well-controlled thirty-day study of marijuana users (Jones & Benowitz, 1976). Tolerance to endocrine system alterations, cardiovascular changes, and sensual effects developed at different rates; tolerance did not develop at all to some of the endocrine system alterations measured. Some of the sensual drugs may not seem to be associated with tolerance or withdrawal symptoms; however, I have observed that extended use usually leads to some degree of chemical addiction.

Scientists used to think that marijuana, cocaine, and the amphetamines were not chemically addictive. They observed some behavioral changes when the use was discontinued, but they considered these to be physical symptoms of emotional stress and evidence merely of a psychological dependency. Only opiate withdrawal symptoms were considered signs of a real addiction. We now know that each sensual drug has its own characteristic withdrawal symptoms whose severity depends on the degree of the drug's effect on the nervous system and the rate at which it leaves the body. In the past several years, experiments have indicated that chemical addiction occurs to some degree with all the sensual drugs. The characteristics of chemical addiction for each of these drugs are discussed below.

Marijuana

When the user begins to take marijuana, he at first sees no evidence that he is building up a tolerance. Usually he experiences no effects the first few times he uses the drug. Then, the first time he becomes intoxicated, he finds, for a time, that even smaller amounts have an effect. The heightened sensitivity of the new user has several explanations:

1. Many beginners do not smoke enough to get the maximum effect. The user must learn to draw the smoke deep into the lungs and hold it there for several seconds.

2. The effects of the initial, usually low, doses are subjective and subtle. Those who describe smoking low-grade marijuana often state that the
beginner may have to learn to discern and appreciate the subtle sensations.

3. Most significantly, THC accumulates in the body. It has been.
found that marijuana metabolites remain in the body for months and
that radioisotope-labeled THC persists in the brain.

For a detailed discussion of the accumulation of THC in
the body, see Appendix 2. Here, a brief summary is
provided.

The cannabinols are unique among the sensual drugs in
their capacity to be absorbed and retained in the lipid (fat)
structures of brain cell membranes and the fat cells of the
body. They have an extraordinarily high fat/water solubility
ratio – approximately 6000 : 1, compared with 300 : 1 for
most intoxicants. Marijuana's high fat solubility and inability to be metabolized account for its long retention time
and for the immediate and persistent effects. In a similar but
not identical way, the salts of mercury and lead accumulate
in the body over time. Their presence eventually causes
muscle tremors, insomnia, confusion, restlessness, irritability, and headache.

THC is absorbed from the blood into the brain and other
organs that have a high blood flow – gonads, heart, liver,
and lungs. For some unknown reason it takes several exposures before the brain can absorb enough THC for any
effects to become apparent. Then, because of the accumulation of THC in the brain, reverse tolerance occurs, and
even smaller amounts can produce a high. When the brain
chemistry has sufficiently compensated for its burden of
THC, the doses must be increased to obtain a high. At this
point, the user has built up a tolerance to THC. With each
high, the blood, brain, and other organs experience a transitory increase in THC concentrations. The amount declines
slowly over four to six hours as THC in the blood is dumped

into body fat. During this time, the THC levels in the organs remain in balance with the THC level in the blood. Small amounts of THC are excreted in urine, and larger quantities leave the body by way of the bile into the feces, but most THC is absorbed from the blood by the body fat, where it is retained; the accumulation increases with each new exposure. THC is resorbed slowly from the fat into the blood when the level of THC in the blood drops. In this manner, low concentrations of THC are recycled to the brain and other organs, and small fractions are excreted in the feces. Briefly, then, fatty tissue acts as a storehouse for THC. The marijuana high is produced by the THC that goes to the brain immediately after exposure; the THC stored in body fat, which comes back into circulation as the blood level of THC drops, accounts for the persistent effects. Months of abstinence are required for all the accumulated THC to be excreted from the body.

That tolerance to THC develops has now been well established. One researcher has said: "Hashish smokers I have known for twenty years are now able to smoke at least ten times as much as other people. If a beginner smoked the same quantity he would collapse" (Miras, 1970). Another has pointed out that perhaps the best evidence for the development of tolerance to marijuana comes from the La Guardia Report, which indicated that the dose required to produce ataxia was three times greater for users than for nonusers (Paton, in U.S. Senate Hearings, Part V, 1972). From my interviews, I have found that casual smokers are satisfied with low-potency marijuana cigarettes, but that experienced, regular users smoke more when they have cigarettes of low potency and less when they get cigarettes containing more THC. The casual smokers who use high-potency cigarettes are often severely affected or at least have unpleasant effects.

According to their tolerance, daily users smoke between 8

and 60 milligrams of THC per day. American soldiers both in Germany and in Vietnam escalated to very high doses of THC when the supply was almost unlimited.

Direct evidence indicates that tolerance to THC also develops in animals. Pigeons are good subjects for experimentation because they can be trained to peck at keys for food according to a complicated schedule. The pigeons used in one study (McMillan *et al.*, 1970) were given doses of THC high enough to suppress all pecking activities. After five days at this level, they began pecking as much as they had before. The dose was then increased to a level twenty times that of the original dose. The pecking stopped, but after twenty-seven days at this level, the pigeons began pecking as before.

Until recently, although tolerance was recognized, marijuana was not considered a chemically addictive drug because of the mildness of its withdrawal symptoms. New information about how THC accumulates and is retained in the brain and body fat explains the mildness of the withdrawal symptoms in terms of dose and distribution of THC in the body. A person who has taken large doses of THC for a short time experiences the most marked withdrawal symptoms. His brain mechanisms adjust in one or two weeks to a high dose. When this happens before the stored levels of THC approximate the peak blood levels (a process that takes many months) and marijuana use is then stopped, there is a great difference between the peak levels in the blood (to which the brain's tolerance has become adjusted) and the stored levels. The blood does not pick up enough stored THC from the body fat to meet the brain's tolerance demands. When the brain's controls cannot obtain the high level of THC to which they are adjusted, withdrawal symptoms appear. In the chronic user, the peak levels of THC in the blood and brain are nearer the stored levels. His withdrawal symptoms are mild because his blood draws on stored THC to meet his brain's tolerance-adjusted demands. During the first week of abstinence (following long-term exposure), he has essentially no withdrawal symptoms; subsequently, he experiences only low-grade symptoms.

Other sensual drugs produce more marked withdrawal symptoms because they are not stored in the body. Undoubtedly, if THC were expelled from the body as rapidly as other sensual drugs, it, too, would produce intense withdrawal symptoms in the chronic user.

Like tolerance, withdrawal symptoms have been observed experimentally in both animals and humans (Kaymakçalan, 1973). Cats and rats showed behavioral disturbances amounting to withdrawal symptoms when regular administration of THC was interrupted. Rhesus monkeys show symptoms closely resembling those of humans. In one experiment, six rhesus monkeys were given THC four times a day for twelve days. At first the monkeys could not be trained to press levers in their cages to give themselves intravenous injections of THC solution. The monkeys were apparently not experiencing pleasurable effects. However, in the second experiment, after the involuntary injections were stopped, all six monkeys had definite withdrawal symptoms, and two out of six then took up regular patterns of self-administration. After that, each time the monkeys were exposed to regular doses of THC that were suddenly terminated, they developed withdrawal symptoms. The abstinence syndrome consisted of hyperirritability, increased aggressiveness, tremors and muscle twitches, yawning, photophobia, and erections in the males. The intensity of the symptoms varied among the six monkeys tested, but their behavior was similar; the monkeys pulled their hair, bit their fingers, ate unusual things, stared, and grasped at imaginary objects (Kaymakçalan, 1972, 1973).

In humans, marijuana withdrawal symptoms typically

appear in the form of reversed effects – irritability, restlessness, and sleeplessness. However, more intense withdrawal symptoms have been observed in persons exposed for a few weeks to high doses of THC (210 milligrams daily) (Jones & Benowitz, 1976). The experiment employed volunteers who were already marijuana users. Because of the various levels of THC already accumulated in their bodies, the time required to build up tolerance to this high dose and the intensity of the withdrawal symptoms would be expected to vary. This proved to be the case. At the beginning of the experiment, some subjects reported severe intoxication, and others reported little or none. Those who were at first numbed by the high doses later had only minimal effects when administered the same dose. The intensity of the withdrawal symptoms also varied. They included restlessness, sleeplessness, rapid onset of irritability, loss of weight, nausea and vomiting, diarrhea, increased salivation, sweating, hot flashes, runny nose, hiccups, and electroencephalographic changes during sleep.

Although 210 milligrams of THC is about ten times greater than the usual dose in the United States, some marijuana smokers use more. A United Nations survey showed that in some cultures 500 milligrams is commonly used daily. A survey of American soldiers in Germany showed that many took as much as 200 grams of hashish (containing 10 percent THC) per month (equal to about 600 milligrams of THC per day) (Tennant, in U.S. Senate Hearings, 1974). In another study some subjects voluntarily used up to 200 milligrams of THC per day (Mendelson *et al.*, 1974*a*). A critical scientific review of the Mendelson study states: "Any assertion that cannabis is a drug which cannot produce tolerance is, after this study, certainly no longer credible" (Edwards, 1975). (Marijuana available in the United States ranges from 5 to 140 milligrams of THC in a 1-gram cigarette. A so-called 1 percent cigarette weighs 1 gram and contains 10 milligrams of THC; a 2 percent cigarette weighs 1 gram and contains 20 milligrams of THC. The 2 percent cigarettes and those containing more THC are considered "good grass" by marijuana users.)

Marijuana withdrawal symptoms are also noted outside the clinical setting. Mild to distressing symptoms have been reported to me by the marijuana users I have interviewed who gave up the drug. Acute symptoms of marijuana withdrawal were reported in five persons whose supply of marijuana had run out while they were traveling through the African desert. The attending physician noted their anxiety, restlessness, acute abdominal cramps, nausea, sweating, increased pulse rate, low blood pressure, and muscular aches. He later diagnosed these as marijuana withdrawal symptoms when he realized they had disappeared when a courier bringing a new supply of marijuana arrived from the nearest seaport (Bensusan, 1971).

The accumulating evidence that tolerance and withdrawal symptoms occur with marijuana use indicates that marijuana is an addictive drug. The Drug Committee of the World Health Organization concurs and has stated that cannabis falls under its definition of an addictive drug.

Amphetamines

Amphetamine dependency has also been misunderstood. Until recently, it was thought that amphetamines were not chemically addictive. They seemed to create no tolerance to their effects, and the depression, fatigue, and voracious appetite experienced during abstinence were considered merely natural reactions to the hyperactivity, loss of appetite, and sleeplessness of the amphetamine intoxication.

We know now that tolerance can be developed to amphetamines. It develops slowly, but eventually amounts many times the safe limit for the inexperienced user can be ingested.

That tolerance develops was demonstrated in a study of

the electroencephalographic and electrooculographic patterns during sleep of six women who were abusers of amphetamines. The experiment involved a comparison of their brain waves and eye movements with those of non-drug-using adults. During withdrawal, the patterns for the six amphetamine users were altered and required from three to eight weeks to return to normal. When the drug was restored, the return to a normal pattern of brain waves and eye movements during sleep was immediate. By definition, addiction means that some physiological functions that are normal in the addict become abnormal in withdrawal and return to normal when the drug is administered again. The experimenters thus concluded that their patients were physically dependent on amphetamines (Oswald & Thacore, 1963).

The abstinence syndrome of Preludin, a commonly used amphetamine, is characterized by anxiety, a dry mouth, extreme restlessness, nervousness, and sometimes a marked twitching of the fingers, extremities, or even the head (Louria, 1968). The symptoms are relieved by taking more Preludin.

Symptoms of withdrawal from amphetamines tend to be mild. One researcher has suggested that this is because the drug is eliminated relatively slowly from the body (Kalant, 1966).

Cocaine

Soon after its introduction into the United States and Europe in the late 1800s, some physicians advocated cocaine as a wonder drug that could cure everything from tuberculosis and indigestion to morphine addiction. It was used in patent medicines and carbonated beverages, and many people inadvertently became addicted to cocaine. Today in the United States, cocaine is rarely used medicinally and is illegal for most other purposes. Recently large numbers of drug users have started sniffing coke. In 1973 a government study concluded that cocaine was being used at least as widely as heroin and estimated that 4.8 million Americans had tried it.

Cocaine is the principal active ingredient in the coca plant. Although it was isolated over a century ago, its properties have not been investigated as thoroughly as those of the other sensual drugs. It is classified as a narcotic for legal purposes, but pharmacologically, it is a stimulant, not a narcotic. Cocaine acts on the body, not like the opiates, but more like the amphetamines; and weight for weight, it has about the same degree of effect on the nervous system.

Cocaine has a strong sensual impact. However, because the withdrawal symptoms are not like those of the opiates, it has been called only psychologically addictive. Also, many users do not take cocaine often enough to build up tolerance or to have withdrawal symptoms when they stop – primarily because of the nature of its effects and its high price. The pleasurable effect from a dose of cocaine (one snort in each nostril) wears off in less than an hour. It is followed by several hours of nervousness and depression, so that the user must take another dose to maintain his high. Chronic, frequent sniffing is rare because the user reaches such a state of excitement that he voluntarily seeks sedation. In my sampling of college students, none of those who said they used cocaine when it was available was chemically addicted. With chronic use, both experimental animals and humans develop a reverse tolerance or an increased sensitivity to the effects of cocaine. Animals do not appear to develop a regular tolerance to cocaine, and this has led some researchers to conclude that humans also fail to develop a tolerance. However, tolerance and reverse tolerance are entirely separate conditions, and the development of one does not exclude the development of the other.

In fact, through the medical history of the drug, it has been recognized that individuals who use cocaine chronically develop a tolerance that requires increasingly large doses to produce a kick. Most recently, a study reported that the craving for cocaine may be extreme (Caldwell & Sever, 1974); that the tolerance produced is very great; that large doses, up to 10 grams per day, may be taken; and that interruption of use does not reduce the developed tolerance, which is very difficult to lose.

The ability of an individual to tolerate increasing doses of cocaine, and, after several weeks of abstinence, to tolerate the same large dose is explained by the fact that the liver increases its supply of cocaine-destroying enzymes. Larger doses of cocaine are then required to produce the anticipated effects. Once the enzyme balance of the liver has shifted, the condition persists so that even after months of abstinence a high tolerance remains. Humans vary in their ability to build up tolerance to cocaine. Laboratory animals generally have less ability to generate the cocaine-destroying enzymes and, therefore, show little or no buildup of tolerance.

Reverse tolerance, on the other hand, is caused by the buildup of the sensitivity of the brain nerve cells to cocaine. Cocaine seems to irritate the brain cells, causing some of the brain's functions to become hyperactive. Cocaine augments the action of the sympathetic nervous system by preventing or slowing the destruction of the neurotransmitter substance of the sympathetic nervous system, noradrenaline. Chronic use of cocaine causes progressive changes in the relay centers of the autonomic nervous system located in or near the limbic area, the center of sensory pleasure. These deep relay centers show heightened and prolonged electrical (brain wave) activity. Further exposure to cocaine causes the hyperactivity to spread from one nerve relay center to another. Thus, the brain cells become sensitized, and the same dose of cocaine used repeatedly produces increasingly greater behavioral and toxic effects. Reverse tolerance to these effects has then developed.

The augmentation of brain wave signals from the deep brain relay centers can trigger grand mal convulsions in an epileptiform seizure. Cocaine causes chemical changes in the brain's relay centers, indicating that these nerve centers have been chronically irritated.

The reaction of the chronic cocaine user to withdrawal is very much like that of the amphetamine addict; the individual feels hungry, sleepy, fatigued, and depressed. Just as with amphetamines, it was once believed that these symptoms were merely reversed responses to the hyperactivity of cocaine intoxication. Now it is recognized by many authorities that these are true withdrawal symptoms, which disappear when more of the drug is taken. Resumed use of the drug not only eliminates withdrawal symptoms, but also starts a new cycle of use.

But even though psychological addiction to cocaine appears to be stronger than the chemical addiction, cocaine is still a dangerous drug, for two reasons: (1) the two kinds of addictions cannot be separated, and (2) psychological dependency is a powerful force. Though many people seem to be able (so far) to use cocaine moderately, the number of heavy users is increasing.

Cocaine is a potent vasoconstrictor, and sniffing interrupts the supply of blood to the mucous membranes. Repeated sniffing irritates and eventually destroys the membranes that line the nasal passages and sometimes even perforates the nasal septum. Cocaine is readily absorbed through the very nasal mucous membranes it destroys.

Although sniffing is the most usual means of administering cocaine, intravenous injection is also common, especially among opiate addicts. The simultaneous injection of cocaine and an opiate is referred to as a speedball.

Hallucinogens

The repetitive use of any of the powerful hallucinogenic drugs – psilocybin, mescaline, or LSD – causes a rapid buildup of tolerance, which indicates that they are potentially addictive. Dependency on one of these drugs, however, does not usually result because they are used sporadically and seldom on a daily basis. The impression of a powerful hallucinogenic experience lasts for several days or even months; during this time, the user rarely feels the inclination to repeat the experience. Although chemical addiction is thus avoided, marked tolerance does develop if the drug is taken as often as once a week, and the dose must then be increased to maintain the effects. When this happens, most LSD users simply stop for several weeks until their capacity to respond returns.

Alcohol

Tolerance to alcohol develops with frequent use. How fast it develops depends on the pattern of abuse: heavy regular drinkers can consume two to three times more than the novice without feeling nauseous and incapacitated. The level of tolerance is often difficult to ascertain because alcoholics learn to disguise their intoxication. In the late stages of alcoholic cirrhosis, the level of tolerance declines; the liver, whose enzymes break down the alcohol, has deteriorated. In advanced cirrhosis, alcohol cannot be removed from the blood efficiently, and even one drink is enough to produce long-lasting behavioral disorders.

The symptoms of alcohol withdrawal range from confusion to the frightening hallucinations of delirium tremens and are marked by major disturbances of the vital functions. The symptoms have long been recognized, but not until recently was it also understood that they are not just the result of nutritional deficiencies or of the toxic effects of alcohol on the brain. Even when diet is controlled, a characteristic abstinence syndrome can occur after only a few weeks of heavy drinking. Severe withdrawal symptoms, however, do not usually appear until after several years.

With the increase in use of sensual drugs, consumption of alcohol has increased markedly among the young. Drug users like the compounding effects alcohol produces. Also certain drugs, notably marijuana and barbiturates, condition the mind so as to diminish the protective reflex of vomiting. Marijuana and barbiturate users are thus able rapidly to enlarge their tolerable consumption of alcohol. Additionally, those attempting to give up other drug use generally increase their consumption of alcohol. Because alcohol is legal, has been used for centuries, and is readily available, many consider it a mild drug. However, alcoholism, cancer, and cardiovascular and cerebrovascular diseases are the nation's four top health problems. Alcoholism has increased to such an extent among the young that Alcoholics Anonymous now sponsors special groups just to help young alcoholics.

Volatile solvents

Lacquer thinners, solvents in plastic glues, petroleum fluids (such as paint thinners, gasoline, and kerosene), propellants in spray cans (mainly freons), and alcohols (mainly methyl) are the solvents most commonly sniffed for their sensual effects. Compared to other sensual drugs these are easily obtainable and relatively inexpensive. (Although ether has been abused in the past for its sensual effects, due to its cost and unavailability, ether is not commonly used in the present epidemic of solvent sniffing.) The sniffing of solvents has become a global problem. An international symposium on the subject held in Mexico City, June 1976, reported that solvent sniffing is practiced in many countries by boys and girls from five to sixteen years of age and that the practice is rapidly spreading among adults. Because volatile solvents are readily available, controlling their abuse is difficult to impossible. Although Japan kept its drug abuse problems contained in the past, presently it has an epidemic of youthful solvent sniffers – mainly sniffing plastic glues.

Typically the solvent is poured or sprayed into a rag, balloon, or plastic bag and the volatile gases sniffed. Frequently solvents are inhaled through the mouth. Such sniffing was originally reported to be relatively harmless physically; the general impression was that deaths from sniffing resulted from suffocation. Although there is the risk of suffocation from a lack of oxygen in the bag or rag, many solvent sniffers have died suddenly and unexpectedly from heart arrest without suffocation as the cause. It has now been established that volatile solvents are highly toxic when inhaled. Loss of appetite, anemia, and damage to the brain, bone marrow, kidneys, and liver have been reported from the chronic use of these solvents.

Volatile solvents, like anesthetics, are absorbed directly and quickly into the body through the lungs. Dizziness and suppression of mental functions occur. Because of their sensual effects, in this text the volatile solvents are classified as intoxicants; their effects are similar to those of alcohol but they come on more swiftly and the period of intoxication is shorter – in some cases lasting only a few minutes. Unlike alcohol, these solvents are not metabolized but are lost from the body by ventilation from the lungs. Because they are fat soluble, they are held for a time in the body fat; odoriferous solvents can be detected in the breath for many hours after exposure. Tolerance is built up to the sensual effects, but the margin of safety between the dose needed for sensual effects and the dose that causes fatal anoxia is always small. A habitual user of volatile solvents may have a persistent cough from inflammation of his respiratory tract. He may also have a ring of inflamed skin around his nose and mouth from their exposure to irritating vapors. Many chronic sniffers of solvents become chronic alcoholics or barbiturate addicts.

Nicotine

Nicotine tolerance can easily be recognized in the difference between the reactions of a first-time smoker and someone who has a habit. Nicotine causes an oversecretion of hydrochloric acid in the stomach and changes in the intestines, so that a first-time smoker is likely to vomit. He may be dizzy and feel tingling sensations, and his thought may be fuzzy for a few moments. These are symptoms of nicotine's effects on the central nervous system that disappear with continued use. As tolerance develops, the senses of taste, smell, and touch become dulled and insensitive; the smoker can increase his intake of nicotine without feeling any new sensual effects or any nausea and tense nerves. Withdrawal symptoms include restlessness, sleeplessness, and irritability, and are often accompanied by headaches. Many former smokers suddenly gain weight – not because cigarettes helped keep their weight down, but because withdrawal produces a nervous compulsion to eat.

Barbiturates and opiates

No one questions that both the barbiturates and the opiates are highly addictive. Tolerance to the barbiturates develops to the point of dependency in weeks or months. The dose cannot be increased to match the level of tolerance, however, because the lethal dose is low. Since there is little margin of safety, the chronic user is as susceptible to the fatal overdose as the novice. Symptoms of barbiturate withdrawal are similar to delirium tremens. They are more severe than those produced by the other sensual drugs and often result in death.

Tolerance to the effect of opiates can build up as rapidly as the user chooses to increase his dose. Apparently most users increase the daily dose by about 1 milligram of pure heroin. Others build up rapidly, increasing the dose by as much as 10 milligrams. The user tends to level the dose at 300 to 400 milligrams because of the cost and because of secondary complications such as extreme constipation. Unlike tolerance to barbiturates, tolerance to opiates increases the margin of safety; the lethal dose is relative to the tolerance level and increases as tolerance increases. Symptoms of opiate withdrawal are unpleasant, but are certainly bearable and rarely fatal. (See Appendix 3 for more information about opiates.)

Tranquilizers

Tranquilizers are classified as either major or minor. Major tranquilizers, such as the phenothiazines, are used medically for treating mentally disturbed patients. They are not used for their sensual effects. The minor tranquilizers, used to reduce anxiety, include different kinds with slightly varying effects. The ones most commonly employed for their sensual effects in the United States are chlordiazepoxide (Librium), diazepam (Valium), meprobamate (Miltown and Equanil), and glutethimide (Doriden); trade names vary in different locations. The minor tranquilizers produce some of the same psychological effects as barbiturates and alcohol: relaxation, a feeling of well-being, and some lessening of inhibitions. At high doses, the effects are not much different from the effects of barbiturate and alcohol intoxication. How tranquilizers produce their effects is unknown, but like alcohol and barbiturates, they are addictive at high, regular doses.

Tolerance is developed to the minor tranquilizers, and their withdrawal symptoms, similar to each other, are also similar to those of alcohol and barbiturates. As is true for barbiturates, no tolerance develops to the lethal toxicity, and overdose is easy. The abstinence syndrome from abrupt withdrawal can be severe and may cause death.

Cross-tolerance develops for the minor tranquilizers and to the other intoxicants. Different minor tranquilizers may be combined with each other or with other intoxicants to give a variety of sensual effects or to sustain intoxication. However, alcohol and barbiturates taken simultaneously with large doses of tranquilizers may produce toxic or fatal reactions. As tolerance develops, opiate addicts often use large quantities of minor tranquilizers or barbiturates.

Nonsensual use of drugs and addiction

Most users of sensual drugs are introduced to drugs by their peer groups, but some are introduced through prescribed medications. When any psychoactive drug, even though initially taken for medical purposes, is used for its sensual effects frequently and regularly enough – so tolerance builds up and withdrawal symptoms appear when drug use is discontinued – it becomes addictive.

Approximately 1 adult in 500 who is given opiates (other than codeine) as a medication becomes addicted. Physicians are cautious about giving opiates (morphine, Demerol, etc.); when pain-relieving medications are continued longer than necessary, the patient may become conditioned to the euphoria and demand more opiate. The fact that hospitals routinely administer pain-relieving opiates increases the danger of addiction from overextension.

Opiates usually do not create dependency as long as they relieve pain (although secondary effects such as impotence may occur). Codeine, an opiate commonly prescribed to relieve mild or moderate pain and tooth or bone ache, is not likely to cause addiction because it is usually given in closely scheduled doses for short periods.

The quantities of pep and diet pills that are prescribed suggest that the number of people at least mildly addicted to amphetamines is large. Those who obtain relief from mild depression from pep pills and who evaluate the experience as positive are likely to repeat it. The use of amphetamines to reduce appetite often leads to addiction (the incidence is noticeably high among women and young girls) because of the regularity with which the drug is taken and the tendency to speed up weight reduction by increasing the frequency or the amount of the dose. In fact, the appetite-suppressing action disappears after about two weeks unless the dose is increased. Large doses of amphetamines cause compulsive behavior. The regular user who increases, either gradually or compulsively and rapidly, the "medical" dose of amphetamines runs a serious risk of becoming addicted.

About 80 percent of the prescribed amphetamines are used by women patients in the United States (Balter, 1968). A study in Newcastle, England, showed that 85 percent of registered amphetamine-using patients were women, usually housewives between thirty-six and forty-five years of age. It was estimated that more than 20 percent of them were habituated or addicted. The most common reasons for taking the drugs were depression, fatigue, obesity, and anxiety (Kalant, 1966). Students or drivers who use amphetamines to stay awake are less likely to continue into compulsive use because their doses remain small and use is confined to the period of need. Such use does not necessarily help accomplishment of the objectives, however. Students who use amphetamines to stay awake to study are often spaced out in the examination. One complained he was not given enough time to finish the examination; in fact, he had written only a few sentences in one hour. Also, amphetamines have been found with the drivers in a number of fatal highway accidents (other circumstantial evidence also implicated the drug) (Kalant, 1966).

Some athletes experiment with drugs, usually stimulants. However, there is no evidence that drugs improve athletic performance. Stimulants have no effect on the speed of nerve conduction or response time; in fact, they impair coordination. The natural stimulant, adrenaline, mobilizes reserves of energy at the right moment. Stimulants mimic the effect of adrenaline, but they are administered at the wrong time – before the competition begins. This premature mobilization wastes energy reserves by using them before they are needed. The athlete may feel stimulants help him perform better, but his performance is usually less than spectacular. In several studies, urine tests performed on athletes revealed that although the winners had not used stimulants, several of the later finishers had (Cooper, 1972).

A barbiturate used occasionally in small amounts is an acceptable sleeping pill, if used to induce sleep and not to create euphoric sensations; however, tiredness from vigorous exercise produces a natural and more satisfying sleep. With continued use, tolerance to the effects of barbiturates builds up, and the dose must be increased to achieve the desired results. Taken in large quantities, barbiturates are long-acting, and the user finds he needs an amphetamine in the morning, to "counter what is essentially a chemical hangover from the night before" (H. J. Campbell, 1971). This may initiate a pattern of drug use that may lead to serious drug involvement. Another hazard of barbiturate use is that an oversedated user, forgetting he has taken a pill, may take more and achieve an accidental overdose.

Almost 40 percent of all the psychotherapeutic drugs prescribed in the United States are minor tranquilizers. As is true of barbiturates and other psychoactive drugs, regular, frequent use builds tolerance and the dose has to be increased to obtain the desired therapeutic effects. However, the euphoric effects of therapeutic doses of barbiturates and tranquilizers are less pronounced than those of the other commonly used psychoactive drugs. Thus, even though some degree of dependency and tolerance occurs, there is less tendency to progress to compulsive abuse. Tranquilizers and barbiturates are, however, commonly taken by drug users in large doses or in combination with other drugs for the added sensual effects.

Because dependency often develops from the medical use of the psychoactive drugs, these agents should be employed only for relief of immediate distress and only until other treatment becomes effective. Furthermore, they are more effective when tolerance is not allowed to build up.

In many cases of routine, continuous use, it becomes difficult to draw the line between medical use and drug abuse. Physicians have to exercise extreme caution not to overprescribe sensual drugs, not only for the sake of the patient's health, but also lest the drug be given to others as medication or sold for profit. Some patients attempt to obtain prescriptions from several physicians. An ex-addict should not be prescribed a medicine that contains the drug he was formerly addicted to. It is easy for him to become readdicted.

Addiction to prescribed drugs is a hazard, not only for the patient, but also for anyone who has access to the medicine cabinet. The family medicine cabinet is commonly a source of supply for children's surreptitious experimentation with addictive drugs. Barbiturates and tranquilizers are a particular problem, since children quickly increase the dose to get the sensual effects and may overdose or develop dangerous withdrawal complications if the use is interrupted.

Drug use among college males

The percentage of 198 Berkeley male undergraduates (aged from seventeen to twenty-three years) using various drugs is shown in Table 1 (also see Table 9). Alcohol is the sensual drug used by the greatest number of male college undergraduates; marijuana is second on the list. Twice as many male college students smoke marijuana as tobacco. LSD use is high. In my surveys before 1972, I found no evidence of cocaine use among university students. Since 1972, as Table 1 shows, cocaine use has increased rapidly. In 1972, 9 percent of college men had tried cocaine; according to my

Table 1. *Drug use among male college students, 1975–1976*

Drug	Subjects using drugs (%)
Alcohol	80
Marijuana	76
Coffee	71
Tea	68
LSD[a]	41
Amphetamines[a]	38
Cocaine[a]	35
Hashish[a]	34
Tobacco cigarettes	30
Tranquilizers[b]	27
Barbiturates[a]	19
Opiates[a]	19

[a] Used solely by current or former marijuana smokers.
[b] Medical use prescribed for anxiety, tension, and insomnia – largely to marijuana smokers.

latest survey in 1975 – 1976, one in three have tried it. Few students reported use of hashish before 1971; in 1976, 34 percent of those in my sample have used it.

The use of marijuana increased rapidly among college students between 1965 and 1970. The use has gone up slowly since 1970, but it was already high in 1971 (about 70 percent of college males). In addition, the frequency of use and the strength of marijuana have increased greatly since 1971, and users have progressively begun at an earlier age.

The figures cited in Table 1 are for the use of a drug one or more times. The illegal drugs, except marijuana, were probably mainly used experimentally or only occasionally. What percentage of college males were addicted to drugs was not determined. This was determined, however, for soldiers in Vietnam at DEROS (date eligible for return from overseas) from urine sample analysis and follow-up studies (see Chapter 7). The important finding of this follow-up study was that many men were able to give up their drug use voluntarily. This was true even for heroin users, especially those who had smoked heroin less than six months. For further statistics and a discussion of drug use in the United States see the appendix to the U.S. Senate Hearings (1975).

Drug use among patients in U.S. federally financed treatment centers

Drugs used by 41,873 patients admitted to federally financed clinics in the United States are shown in Table 2 (see Appendix 4 for source and further discussion). The figures are based upon reports from treatment centers in thirty-one cities in the United States between January 1, 1974, and March 31, 1975. Some 74 percent of the centers reported. Of the patients included in the report, 13 percent were

Table 2. *Drug use among patients in federally financed treatment clinics, 1974–1975*

Drug	Patients regularly using drug (%)[a]	Patients admitted for use of this drug (%)
Opiates	65.5	55.2
Marijuana	38.0	16.8
Alcohol	19.0	7.2
Barbiturates	16.0	5.1
Amphetamines	13.0	4.6
Cocaine	10.1	1.1
LSD	9.6	3.0
Tranquilizers	5.5	2.1
Solvents	1.7	1.1
Others	0.7	2.5

[a] Some patients used more than one drug.
Source: Data from U.S. National Institute of Drug Abuse (1975).

under eighteen years old; 46 percent were between eighteen and twenty-five; and 40 percent were over, twenty-five. About 73 percent were male and 53 percent were white.

A study of the data reveals several interesting facts. Opiate users run a high risk of developing serious health problems. This is demonstrated by the fact that although more people in the United States use alcohol and marijuana than opiates, opiate use accounts for the greatest number of admissions to drug treatment centers. The figures also show that marijuana use ranks next to opiate use as the reason given for admission, and that two and a half times more people come for treatment of marijuana-associated problems than for alcohol-associated problems. The small percentage of people admitted for cocaine use probably reflects the fact that cocaine sniffing has only recently been increasing in the United States. It may be several years before the clinical findings reflect the recent rapid rise in its use.

Rate of addiction

The degree of dependency and the rate at which it develops are influenced by the potency of the drug; the size of the dose; the duration and frequency of use; and the health, mental state, and age of the user. Although it is difficult to pinpoint precisely when drug use becomes compulsive and frequent enough to constitute dependency, the following estimates have been made of the length of time drug use can continue before dependency is established:

Tobacco
Five years, starting with use of one cigarette per day
One year, starting with five cigarettes per day
One or two months, starting with one pack per day
Marijuana
Of users eighteen to twenty years old who start with occasional use, 30 percent escalate to daily use within three to five years.
Two weeks of daily heavy use
Alcohol
Of those who become addicted, thirty years, starting with occasional use
Ten to thirty years, starting with daily repetitive use
Two weeks of continuous drinking
Barbiturates
One to two weeks, starting with daily sensual use
Two weeks of nightly use of sleeping pills
Tranquilizers
One to two weeks, starting with daily sensual use
Opiates
Six months, starting with occasional use
One month, starting with heavy use
Ten days, starting with daily use
Amphetamines, cocaine
Two uses, starting with doses producing hallucination; dependency and withdrawal symptoms may result from a single use

Failure to understand the persistence of both chemical and psychological dependencies has sometimes led to an oversimplification of the problem of rehabilitation. Because frank withdrawal symptoms are of short duration and can be more objectively measured than psychic upsets, drug dependency is often explained in terms of withdrawal symptoms, and recovery programs are based on their disappearance. In reality, the reversal of psychic conditioning and of the depression of gratification mechanisms takes much more time than simple detoxification; drug hunger may last many months or years.

CHAPTER 6

Sexual deprivation

Even though the hazards of drug use are numerous and real, each user thinks he can somehow escape them. His change of life style may not bother him. He can not see his damaged brain cells or recognize that his memory and reason are impaired; and he can ignore most forms of his sensory deprivation. There is one change, however, that he cannot ignore – his diminished sexual capacity. Although the subject is seldom discussed, it is rare to find an addict whose sexual system is functioning fully. In fact, failure of this system is often the most apparent effect of drug abuse.

I do not want to give the impression that sexual dysfunctioning is more important than the other hazards of drug use. It is, however, very important for understanding what happens in addiction; and an understanding of sexual dysfunctioning can serve as an aid in rehabilitation. It can be the window through which a drug user finally sees what drugs have done to him. I have found that when addicts fully understand the source of their sexual deprivation, they become motivated to stop drug use. And by recognizing the problem, they are made aware of other malfunctions.

Furthermore, more is known about sexual functioning than about other brain functions affected by sensual drug use. This knowledge can help the understanding of other

110

forms of sensory deprivation. Also, the degree of sexual deprivation is a good measure of how much the other sensory functions are suppressed. Finally, the loss of sexual capacity is of immediate interest to almost everyone.

Because many drugs produce a sexlike pleasure, there is a close relationship between drug taking and sex. Both sexual and drug-induced sensations command attention and condition the brain to seek repetition of the experience. This is not to say that all drugs produce sexual sensations, but rather that drugs create the same sorts of desires in a habituated drug user as sex does in a normal, sexually active person. That some of the same mechanisms are stimulated by sex and by drugs was dramatically demonstrated in experiments with drug-addicted physician volunteers: drug craving and sexual potency were both reduced by removing 1 cubic millimeter of tissue in the hypothalamic region of the brain (Roeder, 1973).

Drugs cannot substitute for sex, for they eventually deaden sexual sensations. If an individual becomes addicted after maturity, full sexual functioning – the ability to beget or conceive, reach orgasm, and have sexual dreams – can be disturbed; and if an individual is addicted before he is sexually mature, his psychological development is hindered. Although just how these intricate functions are affected is not fully understood, the essential causes are known. But to understand these causes, we must first understand how the autonomic nervous system exercises control over the sexual functions as the individual grows and develops.

Sexual development

The sexual system is essentially a program built into the brain and set to coordinate the many activities necessary for reproduction. Each person has an internal timetable; the reproductive organs and nerves are set at birth to respond to various hormones that the brain releases on schedule. Built into this program are the primitive mechanical functions of the sexual system as well as drives, instincts, and emotions that direct sexual activity.

The sexual system develops in the embryo. Early in embryonic development, the body's cells become differentiated according to their future functions: some form the visual, auditory, or other sensory mechanisms; some form the skin; others the nervous, circulatory, or sexual systems.

All the cells of the sexual system are destined to respond at adolescence to the presence of certain hormones that are released into the bloodstream at the command of the autonomic nervous system. Even though the sexual system is not capable of functioning for reproduction until then, there are often signs of future sexual capacities in the infant. A three- or four-day-old female, for example, may emit a few drops of blood as though she is menstruating. This happens only once and is the result of the extra hormonal boost given by the mother just before birth. The penis of the infant male sometimes becomes erect when stimulated by a full bladder, and if his penis is held, the baby instinctively begins reflex movements, thrusting his pelvis back and forth. Occasionally, the breasts of a newborn infant secrete milk. This is caused by exposure to the mother's milk-producing hormones during the last stages of development in the uterus. Slightly older children often play with their sex organs and at times seem almost aware of their own sexuality. They do not, however, appear to distinguish between the pleasure they derive from touching their genitals and the pleasure of thumb sucking or hair twisting. As the sexual system develops, preorgasmic sensations can be experienced, but true orgasmic sensations cannot be felt until puberty.

Toward the end of childhood, there is a radical change in the hormonal balance of the body, which signals that the sexual system is becoming capable of reproduction. At some unknown signal, the autonomic nervous system triggers the release of a chain of hormones, causing the hypothalamus and the pituitary gland to increase the amounts of sex hormones released from the gonads into the bloodstream.

The adolescent undergoes radical physical and emotional changes. The changes are initiated by new levels of endocrine gland activity, which result in an abrupt spurt of growth and the enlargement of the genitals. In boys, sperm and semen are produced; in girls, the immature eggs present at birth in the ovaries ripen, and the breasts develop. The sex hormones, mainly estrogen and testosterone, in conjunction with other endocrine gland secretions, trigger emotional changes as well. The surge of growth and development and the increased endocrine activity force the adolescent to develop new habits and ideas. Suddenly the adolescent begins to have sexual dreams, and there is a change in his emotional life that is not easily related to his childhood learning experiences.

We do not understand all the complexities of the changes, but we do know that the basal ganglia of the limbic region, where mood is controlled, are reordered. As a consequence, preorgasmic sensations, which were felt throughout childhood, become much stronger, and orgasm becomes possible for the first time. It has just recently been found that radioisotope-labeled female sex hormones accumulate much more densely in several limbic structures than in other parts of the brain. This suggests that mature sexual functioning depends on the influence of hormones on limbic structures.

At puberty, changes in the brain itself occur simultaneously with changes in the body. These changes may, along with the presence of sex hormones, enable the brain to create new hookups in its system of nerve pathways. This accounts for the radical changes in sensations and moods at puberty.

Sexual dreaming and sensations

Both sexual dreaming and sensations are involuntary events that occur with the chemical changes at puberty. Sexual dreaming is evidence of sexual programming in the brain. With the filling of the seminal vesicles, young men (even those naive about sex) start to have sexual dreams, which are often remarkably explicit. These dreams are not necessarily environmentally conditioned, but occur spontaneously and can evoke mentally the full sex act, both the preorgasmic phase and the climax with ejaculation. The penis is usually not erect and certainly is not stimulated; all activity except the final ejaculation takes place in the brain.

Drugs, notably marijuana and the opiates, can diminish the capacity for sexual dreaming, probably by deadening the nerve reflex pathways in the brain that create the dreams. During withdrawal, the heroin addict experiences the equivalent of sexual dreams, but his dreams are about taking heroin. Those withdrawing from addiction to alcohol or tobacco may dream for years of drinking or smoking.

Not only sexual dreaming but sexual fantasies are disturbed by drugs. In a study of 65 adolescent male heroin addicts, researchers found that all the boys experienced "fantasies of omnipotence in the possession of great wealth and power, usually by virtue of owning huge supplies of heroin. Sex and actual acts of achievement are absent in these fantasies" (Zimmering *et al*., 1952).

Changes in the sex organs and functional changes in the brain at puberty join to create new, intensely pleasurable sensations. It is as if there are new hookups in the autonomic nervous system and new pathways to the brain's pleasure centers so that more nerves can connect with the brain and the sex organs. The adolescent has sudden rushes of sexual thoughts. When stimulated, he may lapse into a "hypnotic" state in which the usual thought processes are blanked out. It is as if the brain uses pathways and mental reflexes that have not had time to mature.

Some of the expanded sexual sensations felt in the brain and projected to the erotic areas of the body are the result of the enlargement of the genitals. The penis, clitoris, breasts, and the adjacent tissues enlarge considerably during adolescence. These structures then have more surface area for contact sensations. The sensual nerve endings are stimulated by distended blood vessels in the erected tissues; the clitoris, vaginal surfaces, breasts, lips, and even earlobes fill with blood, giving more pleasurable sensations. It is not known why the erection of such tissues gives such pleasurable sensations, but it may be that sexual sensations are due at least partially to special receptors in the blood vessels. If this is the case, the sensations from these blood vessel receptors are blended with those of the skin.

Autonomic controls of sexual functioning

In addition to controlling sexual programming and emotional responses, the autonomic nervous system controls the mechanical coordination of the sex act. This system, as we have already seen, is composed of two divisions, the sympathetic and the parasympathetic, which perform separate and usually opposite functions.

The mechanics of the sex act involve an intricate relationship between the sympathetic and parasympathetic systems. The sympathetic division dominates the physiological response to excitement, while the parasympathetic controls the calming effects. The first pleasurable sensations of sexual excitement or arousal are linked to a shift to the dominance of the sympathetic nervous system and the release of adrenaline into the bloodstream. During the sex act there is a buildup of tensions in both systems, but the sympathetic dominates the preorgasmic phases. At orgasm, there is a short burst of sympathetic activity followed by a transfer of dominance to the parasympathetic system, which then relaxes the muscles and gives the sense of satisfaction.

The balance of the two systems is evident in areas of the body other than the sex organs: the pupils of the eyes are dilated during the preorgasmic phase and dilate even further just prior to orgasm; then they constrict. Adrenaline and blood pressure rise and fall in relation to the activity of the sympathetic nervous system. Mental activity ranges from excitement, generated by the sympathetic nervous system's controls, to satiation and sleep, as the dominance shifts to the parasympathetic controls at the climax of the sex act.

During intercourse, the body's voluntary and involuntary movements are coordinated in the brain with sexual sensations that reach the level of consciousness. The conscious process in most individuals is a major factor in determining when or if the shift between the two divisions of the autonomic nervous system takes place.

The male orgasm illustrates clearly the complex interaction between the two divisions. Erection, thrusting, orgasm, and ejaculation first involve coordinated action between the body muscles under voluntary control and the smooth muscles of the genital organs under the control of the autonomic nervous system. Control of the voluntary muscles in the sex act entails both learned and reflex adjustment. The adjustments of each movement are coordinated below the consciousness at several different levels of the brain and spinal cord: in the motor centers of the brain stem and the cerebellum, and in the motor nerves of the spinal cord. The body moves to achieve the most pleasurable sensations.

The pleasure is mentally connected with the genitals, but, as with all incoming sensations, the sensory centers of the midbrain correlate the sensations, refine them, then pass them up to consciousness.

Blood flow into the penis is increased both by the action of the sympathetic nervous system, which elevates the blood pressure, and by the action of the parasympathetic system, which enlarges the size of the artery to the penis. During erection, this artery must carry about fifteen times more blood than when the penis is flaccid: Blood flow is also controlled by sphincter muscles in the wall structures of the various vessels. Each smooth muscle is controlled to contract or to relax by the sympathetic or parasympathetic system.

In general, these muscles are so far from being controlled by consciousness that we consider them entirely automatic. The degree of their response, however, is dependent on mood. During the sex act, an individual may learn to control these smooth muscles somewhat by controlling his mood and the events related to mood.

Because parasympathetic nerves control the major sexual responses localized in the genital organs, when these nerves are destroyed in the male, he is unable to achieve erection, orgasm, or ejaculation. In the past, it was assumed that the sympathetic nervous system triggered ejaculation. However, when the sympathetic nerves to the male organs are severed, ejaculation is still possible; erection is weakened, and the mechanisms that block the urinary passage between the bladder and seminal vesicles do not function, so that the semen may be ejaculated into the bladder rather than out the end of the penis. Physicians have been able to retrieve this semen for artificial insemination – a proof that ejaculation can actually take place even though the sympathetic nerve controls are lacking.

Hormones, drugs, and sex

Extensive work has been done on the isolation and identification of dozens of hormones and elucidation of the roles they play in all bodily functions. In the past, assay methods for hormones were complicated and required large quantities of blood. Only recently have simple, quick assay methods requiring only minute quantities of blood been developed. Thus, most past experiments showing the relationship of hormones to growth, development, emotions, or other body functions were limited in scope.

There are at least four sex hormones: estrogen and progesterone, the female hormones; testosterone and androsterone, the male hormones. Each is produced in both males and females. Besides the sex hormones, there are between thirty and forty related steroid substances now identified, and perhaps others yet to be identified, that are controlled and monitored by the autonomic nervous system.

Male and female sex hormones and their related substances dominate in their respective sexes. That is, in the average male, the male sex hormones dominate the reproductive patterns. In males who for various reasons behave as females, a shift in the hormonal balance also occurs, though the shift is never sufficient to invert the biological sex. A female injected with male hormones acquires some masculine characteristics, such as a husky voice, a beard, and some growth of the clitoris. Males respond to female sex hormones by developing breast tissue. Lower animals show even greater hormone-induced sexual shifts. Both the hen and the rooster have residual structures of the opposite sex, and if the natural gonads fail, there can be a complete sexual transformation, including reversal of the reproductive roles, within a short time. In rats, sex hormones injected into the hypothalamus induce male or female behavior depending on the site of injection. For example, when a lactation hormone is injected into a certain area of the hypothalamus in male rats or in virgin female rats, both begin to build nests and take care of young rats.

Sex hormones are used medically in humans and other animals to shift hormonal balance. The contraceptive pill, in which a mixture of estrogen and progesterone is administered to prevent ovulation, is perhaps the best known hormone supplement. In a monthly cycle, when the estrogen level declines, the hypothalamus and the pituitary gland of the female initiate the release of a bud of tissue on the ovary known as the egg follicle. When artificially administered estrogen and progesterone reach the control centers of the brain, the centers react as though the egg were still alive and its follicle producing natural estrogen and progesterone; the pituitary does not release the hormone causing another egg follicle to mature and be shed.

The pituitary's follicle-stimulating hormone, which stimulates the ovaries to mature and release eggs, is used to induce ovulation in women whose infertility seems due to failure to ovulate. This hormonal treatment is often successful, but has one disadvantage: often several eggs are shed at a time. The recent rise in the birth of quadruplets and quintuplets is a result of the use of this hormone. Artificial administration of the hormone does not permit ovulation to quench the hormone level as usually happens through the pituitary, so other eggs continue to be released – an example of how crude artificial administration of a drug is, compared with the normal function.

Hormone supplements are also given to replenish an insufficient natural supply of hormones resulting from castration or aging. In women, the ovaries tend to scar over so that the egg follicles cease to produce estrogen or progesterone. During this menopause stage, the absence of sex hormones causes some wasting of the tissue structures and changes in emotional response. These changes can be prevented or reversed by administering small quantities of the female hormones. Sex hormones are also necessary for muscular and skeletal vigor. Osteoporosis, the wasting of the skeleton, is a common affliction of older people, particularly women. Artificial administration of the sex hormones prevents decalcification of the bones.

The extent to which drugs mimic the action of hormones or depress and stimulate their release into the blood is known in only a few cases. We do know, however, that drugs cause changes in functions that are normally controlled by hormones. It is reasonable to conclude from this that hormones are disturbed by drug use. Studies have shown that long-term use of opiates and marijuana depresses the levels of pituitary gonad-stimulating and sex hormones. Marijuana depresses both types of pituitary gonad-stimulating hormones, causing a lowering of sperm and male hormone production. Enlarged breasts have been observed in some male marijuana users. Heroin produces a persistent depression of the adrenal steroid hormone, cortisone. An excess of this hormone can be responsible for feelings of euphoria; deficiency causes depression. Changes in mood resulting from other drugs correspond to moods induced by hormonal changes. Studies also show that amphetamines stimulate the release of adrenaline from the adrenal glands. Chronic, heavy users of marijuana have dry, scaly skin much like that produced by thyroid hormone deficiency. Opiates disrupt the menstrual and ovulation cycles of many female addicts. Ovulation is depressed by opiates, but it is likely to recur during withdrawal. In women opiate addicts, disruption of menstruation is often misinterpreted as pregnancy. We will probably find that drugs cause other extensive hormonal changes. These, in conjunction with a conditioning of responses, are major causes of the disrupted sexual functioning encountered in drug abuse. Hormonal changes may be a cause of other problems, such as drug hunger and the maladjustment of the brain's controls, that persist long after detoxification.

The adolescent has a difficult time coping with his normal sexual development. The artificial stimulation of his sexual instinct can turn the process of development into a nightmare. Sensual pleasure from the drug tends to dominate the natural sensations, making emotional and sexual adjustments even more difficult.

The difficulty in sexual adjustment experienced by the preadolescent drug user is somewhat similar to the deep psychological trauma of a child who is sexually molested before puberty. The sexual organs mature physically, but the victim sustains deep emotional scars. In both cases, sexual programming in the brain is upset by the combination of psychological and physical disturbances. More extensive blood assay work on drug addicts may eventually show that part of the difficulty experienced by those addicted before puberty is due to hormonal upsets.

Marijuana use by prepubertal males may depress hormone levels and delay the onset or completion of puberty (Kolodny *et al.*, 1974). I have studied three young men, eighteen to twenty years of age, who used marijuana through adolescence. Their sexual development had been disturbed by the drug – they never had sexual dreams, nocturnal emissions, morning erections, or any desire to masturbate. When they gave up marijuana use, they began to develop sexually and within a few months had attained sexual maturity.

Drugs and sexual sensations

In small doses, sensual drugs enhance the sex act; in larger doses, they replace the sensations of the sex act. This is simply the result of their profound effect on the autonomic nervous system. The amphetamines and cocaine stimulate or mimic the action of the sympathetic nervous system, causing the blood pressure and pulse rates to increase, the sexual organs to enlarge and become engorged with blood, and the whole body to rise to a high level of excitement. The mind interprets these effects as preorgasmic sexual sensations. Opiates stimulate or mimic the action of the parasympathetic nervous system and produce sensations the mind perceives as the satiation of orgasm and postorgasm. Barbiturates, tranquilizers, and alcohol do this, but to a much lesser degree.

Most of the drugs taken for pleasure give the user, at least for a time, a euphoric sense of self-confidence and well-being. Confidence is usually a prerequisite to the successful performance of the sex act; and a feeling of relaxed well-being is the dominating sensation of its aftermath. Thus, the drug-induced sensations are similar to the psychological events that normally make sex possible and pleasurable.

Although it is obvious that drug users get some kind of sexlike pleasure from drugs, most of them, when interviewed, insist that there is a distinct difference between drug-induced and naturally induced sensations. Their observations concur with the physiological facts. The sensual drugs affect the brain, the senses, and the mechanisms of the nervous system. The natural channels for transmitting, interpreting, and responding to information going from the senses to the brain are bypassed, distorted, and complicated. The user can feel something akin to sexual sensations, without genital stimulation, without the stimulation of sexual thoughts, and without establishing emotional contact with another person. Those who actually make love while on drugs often admit that "it just isn't the same." This is not surprising since no drug can reproduce the complete sex act: it approximates preorgasmic, orgasmic, or postorgasmic sensations, but cannot coordinate all the systems involved. How a user interprets drug-induced sensations depends on his past experience and the circumstances he associates with pleasurable sensations. One who has never experienced sexual activity, for example, is not likely to describe drug-induced pleasurable sensations in sexual terms.

Drugs and sex

Not all drug users, of course, experience the same patterns of disruption of their sexual functioning or the same degree of sexual deprivation. The health of the user, the length of time he has been using drugs, the dose, the method of administration, and his expectations all make a difference in the response.

The following discussion is based on material gathered from my 1,900 interviews with drug users. Although many drug-induced, pleasurable sensations were described to me, here I will discuss only the sexlike sensations and the effects associated with sexual functioning.

Opiates

The opiates (opium, morphine, heroin, and methadone) deliver intense, pleasurable, and satisfying sensations. However, the opiate user gradually loses both his ability to feel pleasure from other sensations and his capacity to function sexually. The literature on opiate addiction rarely recognizes this effect, but its importance should not be underestimated. Often the hope that the capacity for pleasure and sexual functioning will return is the addict's greatest incentive to go through withdrawal and become rehabilitated.

Sensations from opiates vary somewhat according to type and to the method of administration. In 1700 a London physician, John Jones, in *The Mysteries of Opium Revealed*, described oral ingestion of opium: "It has been compar'd (not without good cause) to a permanent gentle Degree of that Pleasure, which Modesty forbids the naming of" (Judson, 1974).

When an opiate is injected, the sensations are immediate and orgasmic, centering first in the pelvic-pubic area, spreading to include the abdomen, and from there radiating throughout the rest of the body. There is a rush of pleasure. Physiologically, the rush occurs because the opiate acts on or mimics the effects of the transition from the sympathetic to the parasympathetic nervous system, bringing the sense of satiation with sexual climax. These intensely pleasurable sensations experienced after the intravenous injection have been called a "pharmacogenic orgasm" (Chessick, 1960).

Many heroin users have reported to me that, after the effects of the drug have worn off, they feel a general sense of depression and discomfort for several mornings thereafter, even if they have taken the drug only once. This seems to be part of a transitional phase: the malaise is not a symptom of withdrawal, but is a residual, depressant effect of the drug on the sensory correlative control and gratification centers. It is the first evidence a user may have that opiates can have long-lasting effects.

In the next step of the transitional phase (that is, before physical dependency is established), heroin users report that sexual dreams and morning erections, common to most young men, cease and they do not feel inclined to sexual activity. Even some of those who use heroin only a few times and then stop for several days find that even when an opportunity to have sex presents itself, they are unable to have an erection.

Many users who continue to take heroin during this phase discover that the immediate pleasure from the drug is decreasing and that they must increase the dose. As this happens, about half the users suffer from severe sensory depression and lose all interest in sex; the others are still capable of erection and even prolonged sexual intercourse, but are unable to reach climax. Users with this partial sexual incapacitation perpetuate the myth that heroin is an aphrodisiac. Some male prostitutes, for example, who use heroin intermittently report that shooting up with heroin before having sexual relations helps to prolong erection, but impairs the climax.

Users who gradually increase their dose of heroin to the point that they are unable to stop without incurring withdrawal symptoms then find their sexual incapacitation is complete; they cannot get an erection or have a natural sexual orgasm. For these users, taking heroin replaces sex.

The orgasmic nature of heroin injection often disguises from the user his diminishing sexual capacity. Usually, it is not until after he discovers he is hooked on heroin that he also realizes he is impotent. Even then, because of a simultaneous loss of sexual desire, he may not be aware of the change.

It is difficult to pinpoint the actual cause of impotence: the impairment may be due to an incapacitation of either the sensory or the motor reflexes, or it may be the result of a conditioned response of the pleasure mechanism to the drug. In any case, the opiate-induced sensations and the normal sources of sexual sensation must compete for the same gratification mechanisms. The artificial stimulation gradually takes precedence as the mind is conditioned to respond to the drug, and the normal patterns of sexual response lose out.

I have found that when young men addicted to heroin discover their sexual incapacity, they increase the frequency of injection to as many as ten or twenty times a day. Out of a group of eighty heroin-addicted soldiers I interviewed in Vietnam, all reported that they had visited prostitutes before becoming addicted. After they began heroin use, their visits stopped, and they increased their heroin use.

During withdrawal, there can be a brief return of sexual

capacity in the form of dreams, nocturnal emissions, or spontaneous erections, but frequent, involuntary emission of semen in situations unrelated to sexual activity replaces normal ejaculation. An addict sometimes cuts back the dose in order to produce a mild withdrawal that will enable him to have an erection. This, however, is only a temporary side effect of the detoxification process, in which certain aspects of sexual disturbances are temporarily reversed. Actually, impotence is prolonged until rehabilitation is complete.

When seventy former heroin addicts were asked to rate their sex drive, their sex activity, and their enjoyment of sex for the period of time they were taking heroin, most indicated that heroin suppressed all three areas (Wieland & Yunger, 1970). A study of thirty-one adult male heroin addicts found that there was a relative loss of sexuality: the time before ejaculation was considerably longer than normal, and the orgasm was of poor quality (De Leon & Wexler, 1973). In still another study, heroin and methadone users reported "substantial difficulties with many aspects of their sexual behavior and function, particularly delayed ejaculation, impotence, and failure to ejaculate (reach orgasm)." All the heroin users and 95.5 percent of the methadone users reported substantially less desire for sexual activity when they were taking narcotics than when they were drug-free. In addition, the motility of the sperm – the ability of sperm to maintain direction as it swims – was reduced (Cicero *et al.*, 1975).

What has been said about opiates and sex applies to women as well as men. The sensual rush upon injection is the same, and addiction results in the same sensual deprivation. Heroin is often used by women prostitutes to mask their psychological problems. The prostitutes I have interviewed were uninterested in sex and got no satisfaction from sexual activity, although they had experienced normal sexual relations before they became involved with heroin.

These women were as interested as male addicts in regaining their capacity for sexual response.

Amphetamines and cocaine

The stimulants – amphetamines and cocaine – produce sexual sensations that are the reverse of those caused by the opiates. Instead of the pleasurable satisfaction of orgasm, the stimulants increase the sense of excitement associated with preorgasmic sex. Instead of mimicking or acting upon the parasympathetic system, they increase the sympathetic system's production of adrenaline or mimic adrenaline's effect on the nervous system. Stimulants increase and prolong the sense of excitement during intercourse, but they inhibit the transition between the sympathetic and parasympathetic systems and postpone, if not eliminate, the climax. As a result, there is no sense of satisfaction; sexual tension cannot be released.

Stimulant users report intensified sexual feelings, delayed ejaculation, and marathon sexual relations. Women frequently reported intensified sexual fantasy and compulsive masturbation or promiscuity (Angrist & Gershon, 1972). Mann (1972) indicates amphetamines can reverse the order in which the prostate gland and seminal vesicles normally void their secretions during ejaculation. Lewin, who lived from 1850 to 1929, studied preorgasmic stimulation induced by cocaine; he found that cocaine causes "weakness of sexual functions accompanied by augmented erotic desires" (Lewin, 1931)

My recent interviews disclosed that cocaine is preferred over the amphetamines even though it is much more expensive. Users say it gives a more "clear-headed" pleasurable sensation and has more pronounced sexual effects. A questionnaire on the motives for use of six sensual drugs was given to entrants to a U.S. Navy drug rehabilitation facility

(Nail, 1974). Cocaine users gave heightened sexual pleasure as the primary reason for that drug's use. This was given as a reason more often for cocaine than for any of the other sensual drugs.

Cocaine users appear to get the same immediate powerful feelings of sexual excitement from sniffing as amphetamine users get from injecting. Some amphetamine and cocaine users I have interviewed report that, after sniffing cocaine or injecting an amphetamine or cocaine dissolved in water, they ejaculate and feel an orgasmic rush. These sensations may be caused partly by the sexual feelings associated with the injection ritual and partly by the associations of sexual excitement and climax. However, even though the stimulant user ejaculates, his emission does not lead to tranquility and satisfaction, but to further excitement and then frustration. The ejaculation does not result in orgasmic release of tension and loss of erection. When stimulation dissolves into depression, the user is tempted to regain his sense of excitement by taking the drug again. Repeated high doses of cocaine or amphetamines, however, increase the danger of both brain damage and physical deterioration.

Some amphetamine and cocaine users have learned to take depressants, heroin in particular, after they have had several hours of stimulation. The combination is sexlike: the stimulants provide pleasurable excitement, and the heroin produces orgasmic relief. Unlike normal sex, however, the ejaculation, if any, occurs first, when the stimulant is injected, rather than later, when the heroin is injected, even though the latter drug simulates natural orgasm more closely.

Barbiturates and tranquilizers are also used to release the tension of the amphetamine high. Louria, in his book, *The Drug Scene*, describes the pattern of drug abuse in Sweden at the time of his visit during the epidemic abuse of amphetamines in 1967:

During a central-stimulant binge they [the addicts] may remain awake literally for days or weeks at a time, injecting themselves every few hours with increasing doses of Preludin until they develop a tolerance and no longer get an effect. Then, they inject themselves intravenously with a barbiturate, discontinue the central stimulants, fall into a deep and sometimes agitated sleep, finally waking with an abstinence syndrome that results in an intense craving for more Preludin. . . . If they can get more Preludin, they then start on another jag which may again last for many days or weeks. [Louria, 1968]

Stimulants can affect the mechanical aspects of the sex act. They increase both the blood pressure and the tension of involuntary muscles and can abnormally distend erectile tissues. When amphetamines or cocaine are taken before and during sexual intercourse, the user can have several hours of continuous intercourse. He usually cannot reach climax until the effects of the stimulant have subsided. Even then, the climax is not a fully gratifying release of tension because that process is still somewhat depressed by the stimulant. I have interviewed heroin addicts, both male and female, who, unable to become sexually aroused, apply cocaine powder to their genital organs. The drug is absorbed rapidly. The vasoconstrictive action of cocaine closes the venous drainage of the erectile tissue, keeping it filled with blood. However, because cocaine acts as a local anesthetic, sensations from the genital membranes are minimal. There is no orgasm. Erection caused by stimulants can be so intense and the pain so severe (priapism) that intercourse is impossible; the erection can last as long as twenty-four hours (Gay & Sheppard, 1973).

The stimulants are often used as aphrodisiacs by older men who believe they are losing their sexual potency, by young people who simply want to experience greater sensations, and by heroin addicts who want to restore their potency. Heroin addicts sometimes inject a combination of cocaine and heroin for "an added boost" (Winick & Kinsie, 1971). The belief, however, that sexual potency will be restored by using the stimulants is fallacious. Users risk losing whatever sexual potency they have left. The stimulants only make it more difficult to reach orgasm. With the onset of old age, the control mechanisms that effect the transition from the preorgasmic to the orgasmic phase of sexual activity weaken. Sexual arousal, but not climax, can take place.

Actually, when older men have difficulty in becoming aroused, it is not usually because they are physiologically incapable of it, but because they have been conditioned by their previous failures to reach a climax. Although stimulants temporarily cause erection, they do not help the real problem – the inability to reach a climax. In fact, they make it more difficult to have an orgasm and leave the user conditioned for less sexual response than he had before.

For young people, the use of stimulants as aphrodisiacs is particularly hazardous. The stimulants are powerful conditioners, and some can establish psychological dependency with a single dose. The level of sensual excitement is so high that the experience is somewhat like the initial discovery of sex. Drug sensations are not necessarily stronger than those of natural stimulation, but they occur by surprise, without effort, and are novel. It is easy to become conditioned to them.

Stimulants are used by heroin addicts to suppress the unpleasant effects of detoxification and to restore their ability to have an erection. For the detoxifying addict, who has probably not been able to have sexual intercourse for months or even years, getting an erection through stimulants can be very reassuring, even though it actually works against recovery.

The use of stimulants by a detoxifying heroin addict unfortunately makes rehabilitation and restoration of sexual capacity more difficult. He is still capable only of preorgasmic sexual activity, and it is difficult, if not impossible, to have a climax. The stimulant further distorts the pattern of sexual action and satisfaction; the brain has great difficulty restoring the functional balance of its controls. In addition, because of the intensified preorgasmic sensations, the addict may feel the need for a release of tension even more acutely and may resume the use of opiates (or barbiturates or tranquilizers) to relieve the overstimulation.

Stimulants are neither effective aids to rehabilitation nor true aphrodisiacs. Good health is the only effective aphrodisiac. Exercise, proper diet, weight control, and rest will increase both sexual desire and capacity.

Alcohol, barbiturates, and tranquilizers

Alcohol, barbiturates, and tranquilizers are depressants. Although they resemble the opiates in that they activate or mimic the effects of the parasympathetic nervous system, their influence on it is only slight, and their primary effect is to depress the mental processes. Thus, even while these drugs can induce sensations that may increase sexual desire, they also dull the mind, impair coordination, and make the user sleepy – all of which make sexual activity much less likely. Whatever sexual appeal alcohol, barbiturates, or tranquilizers have is probably related to the sense of confidence and well-being they induce. There is no basis to the old myth that they release sexual power, except that they slightly reduce mental tensions. The sex act is rarely enhanced by alcohol, tranquilizers, or barbiturates, and there is a loss of sexual ability with high doses. These drugs are primarily used to release inhibitions.

It usually takes ten to twenty years for alcohol to suppress sexual desires. A loss of potency actually caused by alcohol is often wrongly attributed to the effects of aging. Impotence in old age is not inevitable. For the most part, the loss of sexual interest and capacity in the alcoholic results from the conditioning of his mind to the satisfaction of alcohol and from diminishing the mental and physical vitality on which his sexual ability depends. In the case histories of alcoholics I have studied, impotence followed their alcoholism. Damaged testes have been found in men with histories of alcoholism. It is difficult to know whether the changes in the testes were associated with persistent impotence, the toxic effects of alcohol, or the inability of the liver to neutralize female hormones produced in the male (May *et al.*, 1975).

Marijuana

Many people smoke marijuana for erotic stimulation. They say that it relaxes them in social situations, makes finding a sex partner easier, and increases the tactile pleasure and the duration of the sex act. The effects of marijuana, however, are often unpredictable and highly individual. There is evidence that it can actually interfere with sexual performance. Some individuals have reported that they cannot reach a climax while they are high; others indicate that they cannot even become aroused.

Sensations obtained from marijuana seem to depend to a large extent on the mood of the user, his surroundings, and his anticipation of the effects. In a study of the effects of marijuana on sex, the responses shown in Table 3 were recorded (Goode, 1969).

A sampling of college students found that the subjects who smoked marijuana the most were the ones who had experienced sex with a number of partners and who had had sex early in their lives. It could not be concluded, however, whether sex caused the drug use or drug use caused the sexual activity (Goode, 1972).

A study of 1,238 users of cannabis drugs in India (Chopra & Chopra, 1939) also noted the drug's effects on sexual performance (Table 4).

Table 3. *Effect of marijuana use on sex, American study*

Effect	Subjects reporting effect (%)
No effect on sexual desire	33+
Negative effect	5
Effect depends on sexual partner	13
Definitely increased sexual desire	44
Increased sexual enjoyment	68

Source: Data from Goode (1969).

The variations in the effects of marijuana are not entirely subjective. Marijuana is unique among the sensual drugs in that it can act as a hallucinogen, a stimulant, a depressant, an intoxicant, or a combination of all four.

The effects of marijuana on the sexual mechanisms are complex. Although it is not as powerful as cocaine and the amphetamines, it can cause increased blood pressure, which in turn can intensify the erection of the penis. In some people, it may cause a delay in the shift from the preorgasmic to the orgasmic phases of the sex act so that climax is delayed.

The hallucinogenic nature of marijuana alters sensory information so that all sensations initially seem more intense.

Table 4. *Effect of cannabis use on sex, Indian study*

Effect	Subjects reporting effect (%)
Sexual depression	40
Sexual stimulation	16
Initial stimulation, later depression	20
No effect	24

Source: Data from Chopra and Chopra (1939).

Colors are brighter, sounds are clearer, food is more tasty, and it feels better to be touched. Often the variety of sensations is so engrossing that the individual is not interested in sex at all; but if he does find his attention is turned toward the erotic, this sensory magnification could certainly enhance the experience. The hallucinogenic distortion of time, too, combined with the delay of climax, extends the preorgasmic phase over a much longer time than usual.

Although these effects are very pleasurable to some, others have found that the drug has a debilitating effect on sexual capacity and enjoyment. I interviewed several men who had taken marijuana just before having intercourse and who reported that the drug caused painfully overextended erections. Others reported that when they ejaculated, they had painful anal spasms that lasted for a considerable period. These effects were agonizing enough to make the men temporarily disinterested in sex and certainly not interested in repeating the experience.

I found in questioning marijuana users that sexual dreaming is commonly suppressed or impaired by the drug. Actually, the users were unaware of the drug's effects on sexual dreaming until they stopped taking marijuana. In one young man who withdrew from marijuana, this phase lasted approximately six months. During this time, he was frustrated by sexual dreams in which he could not experience sexual climax. His ability to release sexual tensions in nocturnal emissions slowly returned over about a year's time.

Marijuana is similar to alcohol in that it lessens the will of the user to act independently and to resist suggestions made by companions; this loss of willpower weakens the ability to resist coercion. Marijuana causes a curious disjunction between the individual and his ideas, actions, and knowledge of the consequences; between what his mind thinks and accepts and what he actually does. These effects upset reasoning and sometimes lead marijuana users to become involved in activities they normally would avoid. For instance, approximately one out of every five students who come to me for advice is troubled by a homosexual encounter in which he participated while high on marijuana. The student is disturbed by the episode and seems to feel that the encounter has caused subsequent difficulty in relationships with the opposite sex. It appears that the marijuana user is susceptible to any sexual invitation and lacks the will to resist.

If a marijuana user becomes tolerant of the drug to the point that he must take higher doses or more potent samples, he may find that these larger doses decrease the amount of sensory information the nerves can pick up and transmit. The mental magnification effect fails, and the sensory endings become anesthetized. The sense of touch diminishes in intensity, and those who use large doses actually become quite numb. As a result, although marijuana may enhance sex at the beginning, when taken in small doses, it becomes a progressively less satisfying sexual stimulant. This is one reason the marijuana smoker is likely to try drugs with a stronger sensual effect: he can get more intense mental sensations and less anesthetic effect.

Middle-aged people who feel their sexual powers waning sometimes use marijuana in the hope that it will rejuvenate their sex lives. They probably find that at first it will, like other novelties, enhance desire and make the sex act more exciting. With continued use, however, their pleasure usually decreases, but if they stop using the drug, they may find that they have become conditioned to arousal only with the aid of the drug and so cannot perform without it. If they are willing to try higher doses, the numbing effect increases and they have difficulty in reaching climax. They may blame their difficulties or impotence on advancing age. Many of them, however, could probably recover their physical and mental health with proper efforts.

LSD

This hallucinogen is also a mild stimulant and hence enhances slightly the preorgasmic sensations. However, LSD is rarely taken primarily for sexual pleasure; most users are so distracted while high that they are completely indifferent to sex. The vivid hallucinations and extensive mental disorientations are too confusing to allow the user to concentrate long on anything. As is true of marijuana use, expectation seems to play a role in determining what form the LSD trip will take: if the user expects to have a religious experience, the odds are that he will; if he wants a sexual trip, he will probably have that.

The reports concerning the sexual capacity of a person on LSD vary. Some users say that their sex acts take place in fantasy rather than in reality; some report that they are altogether impotent while they are high; others are able to have intercourse if they wait until the more intense hallucinations have subsided; others report no sexual impairment at all and say their sexual experiences on LSD are very enjoyable. The last group claims that the actual duration of the sex act is increased and that hallucinations magnify the sensations of orgasm. Because LSD is a mild stimulant, it may in some cases intensify erection and delay the shift from the preorgasmic to the orgasmic phase of the sex act. It is not a powerful enough stimulant to block completely the orgasmic phase of sexual activity.

Like marijuana, much of the sexual enhancement of LSD is illusory, apparently arising from the hallucinations and a distortion of the sense of time. At times, psychedelic drugs may create increased sexual enjoyment, but they also decrease physical coordination and concentration (Gay & Sheppard, 1973).

Multiple drug use is so common among those who take LSD that it is difficult to gauge the long-range effects of

LSD on sexuality. Some users report sexual disturbances they attribute to LSD, but these may be the consequences of the stimulant or depressant drugs they also take. Another problem in determining the independent effects of LSD is that extended use of the drug causes mental confusion or mental illness sooner than it disorders sexual function. While the mental confusion may be accompanied by sexual disability, it is impossible to know how much of the effect is due to the direct influence of the drug.

The effect of sensual drugs can be categorized as functional or psychological. Opiates, amphetamines, and cocaine imitate sexual sensations produced by the autonomic nervous system. Marijuana, alcohol, barbiturates, tranquilizers, and LSD alter the psychological events related to sex. In both instances, the brain's program for the sexual system is influenced by the drug.

The emotional changes caused by the so-called milder drugs may be the result of changes in the hormonal balances, which may in turn affect the sexual system.

No one can say precisely how a drug will affect his sexual system. The change may seem at first to benefit the user and enhance his sexual activity, but the sensations are unnatural, and his system will not long sustain them as pleasure. He then has to continue taking drugs just to keep from feeling bad.

The needle and sex

We usually associate opiates with injection, but most sensual drugs can be administered in this way. The sexuality of the drug experience is not limited to sensations induced by the drug itself. Some drug addicts get so great a thrill from the injection procedure that the effects of the drug are completely overshadowed. Administering the drug is a ritual for the mainliner, and the details of the performance suggest that it is meant to symbolize sexual intercourse. The addict first "erects" a vein by cutting off the circulation in his arm with a strap. He fills a needle and its attached tube with a drug, punctures the skin, and eases the long point into the vein. Instead of immediately injecting the drug, he pumps the needle in and out of his arm until he reaches a peak of excitement. He then forces the solution out of the needle and into his arm in short, ejaculatory spurts.

Addicts are quite frank about interpreting the injection in sexual terms. Although it is sometimes referred to explicitly as masturbation, most often the drug world jargon attaches gender and specific sexual equivalents to its various elements. The needle is often associated with the penis, the drug with semen, and the vein with the female organ. Heroin is known as "boy," and the vein is identified by the feminine pronouns. The slang is not always consistent, however, and the genders are sometimes reversed: the distended vein, erected like a penis, is masculine, and the needle and the drug are feminine.

The injection equipment is used to enhance the sensuality of the act. Instead of a regular hypodermic syringe, the addict usually uses an outfit made from an eyedropper fastened to a hypodermic needle. This enables him to inject the drug in spurts and, as part of the thrill, to draw up the blood into the apparatus where he can see it. Although he is aware of the hazard, he often prefers to share a dirty needle. Finally, in order to keep his vein sensually distended, he wears the compression band throughout the procedure. Contrary to what some people believe, he does not do this to protect himself from overdose, but to enhance the sexual effect by controlling the flow of the drug. Often when an addict is found dead from overdose, he still has the tourniquet bound tightly around his arm.

The association the addict makes between the injection of the drug and the sex act reflects a relationship that has its basis in the complexities of human physiology and psychology. The sexual organs of both men and women are composed of a spongelike arrangement of vascular tissue, richly supplied with blood. Erection occurs when the individual is sexually excited. Nerve impulses and the secretion of hormones cause the pulse rate and blood pressure to increase. The arteries leading to the erectile tissue are dilated to admit more blood, while the veins that carry the blood away are constricted. The tissue thus becomes engorged with blood, and the organ becomes stiff and hard. Although much sexual pleasure is derived when the specialized nerve endings in the penis or clitoris are touched, it is enhanced by touchlike sensations that emanate from the distended vessels themselves. Thus, the turgid veins of the arm also give the addict pleasure, which is enhanced by the pricking and pumping of the needle.

The novice does not get a thrill from probing the vein with the needle; for him, injection may be quite painful. It takes a period of conditioning to make the transition from pain to pleasure. Conditioning takes place easily because the painful sensations of the injection are followed by the pleasure of the drug's effects, and the association is quickly set in memory.

One consequence of this conditioning is that although the effect of the drug decreases as tolerance is built up, the addict's response to the needle increases. He finally reaches the point where even a fix of water will bring on a sensual rush and postpone withdrawal symptoms. Addicts have been known to inject cough syrup, alcohol, spices, even peanut butter. This can, of course, be extremely dangerous, for particles of these substances are carried in the bloodstream to the lungs, where they block the absorption of oxygen, causing dizziness or even instant pneumonia. A person may survive such an injection, but his lungs are permanently scarred.

Conditioning to the needle is hard for the addict to break.

For detoxified addicts, just the sight of the needle is enough to trigger mild symptoms of withdrawal – even months after detoxification.

Intravenous injection produces a great impact because a stronger dose can be administered. In the study of American soldiers who used heroin in Vietnam, it was found that those who had smoked heroin longer than six months then tended to inject it because they had developed a tolerance to the amount that could be smoked. Amphetamine users commonly progress from oral administration to injection for the added sensual impact.

CHAPTER 7

Drug abuse among American soldiers in Southeast Asia

Examination of heroin use among United States soldiers stationed in Southeast Asia helps us with the study of drug addiction and rehabilitation in the civilian population.

The use of drugs among soldiers was an extension of the same trend in the United States. The epidemic of drug abuse began in about 1965 in the United States and spread at the same time among the troops in Southeast Asia. There it became a major problem in 1970 and peaked in 1971. At that time, military and civilian leaders were unresponsive to the marijuana epidemic and to the increasing use of amphetamines and barbiturates. However, when large numbers of soldiers began to use heroin, the military was prompt to apply countermeasures. A few months after the recognition of the heroin problem, urine testing programs were established and educational programs against drug use were extended.

A picture of the various aspects of the drug epidemic in the military has been compiled from questionnaires, interviews, and urinalysis data. My observations and samplings of the American soldiers were made in the United States, Germany, Thailand, and Vietnam in 1971, 1972, and 1973.

I had access to unpublished data compiled by Lt. Col. Norman Ream from case histories of 5,000 heroin users and 4,000 nonusers enlisted in the United States Army in Vietnam from September 1971 to September 1972. An official report gives the quantitative data for drug use in Vietnam and after the soldiers returned to the United States. This report, *The Vietnam Drug User Returns* (Robins, 1974), is the source of most statistics cited in this chapter. The 14,000 soldiers studied were in Vietnam during the height of the drug epidemic. They ended their tour of duty on September 1, 1971, and had served in Vietnam an average of twelve and one-half months. More thorough than studies of the civilian population, the reports and data from the armed forces describe an entire cycle of the epidemic, providing factual information on drug use, dependency, and recovery.

Use of heroin

Drug use escalated higher and more rapidly in Vietnam than in the civilian population. From my 1970 sampling at Berkeley, I found that 9 percent of American college men who used marijuana had used opiates at least once. A year later, in October 1971, when narcotics were more readily available, the proportion had increased to 21 percent (15 percent of college men); and by October 1972, it had risen to 40 percent. However, college students tended to use opiates only occasionally. Drug use in the army peaked in 1971, when about half of the marijuana users surveyed had used heroin one or more times. Because opiates were cheaper and more readily available in Vietnam, soldiers who had been in Vietnam for a year were two to three times more likely to use heroin than college males in the United States (Table 5). They also tended to use it more frequently and in larger doses.

The drug culture had already spread in the American

population before the rapid buildup of troops in Southeast Asia in late 1970 and 1971. Robins (1974) states: "Vietnam soldiers did not differ in their pre-service drug experience from a national sample of young men answering a questionnaire concerning their drug use in the same year that most of these soldiers entered service." About 47 percent of the newly enlisted men had been involved with drugs before coming to Southeast Asia, and "the drug (other than alcohol) most frequently used was almost always marijuana" (Robins, 1974). Over half of the marijuana users had also used one or more other drugs. Some 11 percent of the newly enlisted men had already experimented with opiates; 2 percent had used heroin; and about 0.4 percent were addicted to heroin (Table 6). Codeine, taken plain or in cough syrup, was the most common narcotic used before coming to Vietnam.

As civilian drug use increased, each group of newly enlisted men brought more drug users to Vietnam. These drug users converted others, and since potent marijuana, 90 percent pure heroin, amphetamines, and barbiturates were all

Table 5. *Comparison of drug use among American college males and American soldiers, 1971*

Type of drug use	College men using drug (%)	Soldiers using drug (%)
Some use of marijuana[a]	71	69
Some use of opiates (largely heroin)	15	
Some use of narcotics (including heroin)[b]		43
Some use of heroin[c]		34

[a] About 21 percent of college marijuana users had used opiates, largely heroin.
[b] Figures for narcotics are for opiates only; 81 percent of the opiates used in Vietnam was heroin, which was 90 percent pure.
[c] Nearly all soldiers using heroin had also used marijuana; about half of marijuana users had used heroin.
Source: Data on college men from Jones (1971); data on soldiers from Robins (1974).

Table 6. *Drug use among American soldiers in Vietnam who completed duty in September 1971*

Drug	Percent using drugs before Vietnam duty (September 1970)	Percent using drugs during Vietnam duty	Percent using drugs after return to U.S. (May–September 1972)		
			All soldiers	Men who had used narcotics over 6 months in Vietnam	Men self-reporting active addiction at DEROS
Alcohol	99.0[a]	92.0			
No drugs (except alcohol, tobacco, medication)	53.0	30.0			
Any of following drugs	47.0	70.0			
Marijuana	41.0	69.0	45.0		
Marijuana only	17.0				
Marijuana for first time		28.0			
Amphetamines	19.0[b]	25.0	19.0		
Barbiturates		23.0	12.0		
Narcotics	11.0[c]	43.0[d]	10.0	31.0	50.0
Opium (sporadic use)		38.0			
Heroin	2.7	34.0			
Addicted to narcotics (mostly heroin)	0.4	20.0[e]	1.0	4.0	14.0

[a] This figure is taken from N. Ream, unpublished data.
[b] Includes amphetamines and barbiturates.
[c] Largely codeine.
[d] Opiates only (no cocaine use was reported); 81 percent of the opiate used in Vietnam was heroin, which was 90 percent pure.
[e] Includes 9.3 percent detected by urinalysis at DEROS (10.5 percent drug-positive, 1.2 percent not addicted); 7 percent who voluntarily turned themselves in before urinalysis; and 3.7 percent who stopped using narcotics prior to urinalysis at DEROS.
Source: Data from Robins (1974).

cheap and easily available, drug use rapidly reached epidemic proportions. By the time countermeasures were taken against the epidemic in 1971, 70 percent of the enlisted men in Vietnam had used one or more drugs, and 43 percent had used opiates.

I was aware of the use of drugs in Vietnam by American soldiers throughout the late 1960s from interviews I had had with students who were veterans of the Vietnam War. Prior to 1970, returning veterans informed me of the use of strong marijuana (later confirmed), amphetamines, and barbiturates, but they said little about opiate use. By late 1970, however, heroin use was reported to me, and by 1971, epidemic use had made the headlines. By mid-1971, extensive corrective measures had been taken.

On my first visit to Vietnam in September 1971 to aid in the drug rehabilitation program, it was easy to find empty, fingertip-sized plastic vials with plastic screw caps scattered around the grass near the barracks. These vials had contained 0.1- and 0.3-gram quantities of 90 percent pure heroin. Soldiers smoked it by combining it with tobacco in their cigarettes. By my next visit six months later, the vials were no longer being used because they could so easily be detected in clothing. The suppliers were then packaging the heroin in small, flat polyethylene bags with zip closures; these were less likely to be detected. The retail price of 1 gram of this heroin ranged from $3.30 to $12.00 (see Appendix 3, Table 13).

In 1971–1972, the extent of the drug problem was not known because the necessary studies had not yet been completed. Various estimates were made, with some news reports placing narcotics addiction as high as 40 percent. This figure is much too high; drug use is distinct from dependency. Actually, 43 percent of the soldiers had used narcotics while in Vietnam; 34 percent had used heroin. Although the figures show that 38 percent of the soldiers had used opium at some time while in Vietnam, they tended to use it only sporadically, and many were using heroin regularly at the same time. Heroin was the major problem opiate. No cocaine use was noted in Robins's report; therefore, the figures given in the report for narcotics use actually indicate opiate use only. I also found no evidence of cocaine use in Vietnam.

When it became apparent that drug use had reached epidemic proportions, the armed forces personnel set up a urinalysis program. Urine was analyzed for the presence of opiates, amphetamines, and barbiturates. All soldiers were subject to urine testing on the day they were eligible for return from overseas (DEROS). Surprise sweeps – tests at unspecified times and without warning – were also used. Thus, all soldiers were tested at least once, and many twice, during their tours of duty. In field assignments, to reduce necessary facilities, surprise tests were given to one soldier in five. Those in whom opiates were detected were given detoxification treatment.

Urine testing proved effective in reducing the spread of heroin use. Since analysis detects heroin up to three days after use, the military command initially publicized the testing program widely to allow men time to quit use voluntarily. Because the soldiers were not certain what the army's action would be against those with drug-positive urine, the mere threat of the tests caused most of the heroin users who were either lightly addicted or not addicted at all to stop. In 1971, 34 percent of the enlisted men had used heroin. This figure included an estimated 20 percent who had some symptoms of opiate (mostly heroin) addiction (Table 6). Yet a screening of the men at DEROS in September 1971 detected opiate residues in the urine of only 10.5 percent (9.3 percent were addicts; 1.2 percent were not). Before the urinalysis, 7 percent had turned themselves in because they were unable to stop heroin use unaided. It appears, then, that the remaining 16.5 percent had quit in time to have drug-negative urine and that 3.7 percent were addicted at some time while in Vietnam and were included among those who had quit prior to DEROS (used heroin, $10.5 + 7.0 + 16.5 = 34$ percent; addicted, $9.3 + 7.0 + 3.7 = 20$ percent).

Evidence shows that the urine tests were given at a strategic time for those leaving in September 1971. Most had been in Vietnam for about a year (twelve and one-half months on the average); 43 percent used opiates. Those who were using opiates regularly within six months of their arrival in Vietnam were entering the six-month phase of regular opiate use and thus were on the threshold of hardened dependency.

There have been many stories about soldiers avoiding positive urine tests by drinking water to dilute the urine, eating alkaline foods to shift the acidity, exchanging urine samples, or resorting to bribery. Except for a few reported cases, however, I found no evidence that any of these had ever occurred. On the contrary, the evidence indicates that the testing took place smoothly and effectively. It is remarkable that this massive program was implemented so swiftly and carried out with so little error.

The Department of Defense continued urine testing in South Vietnam and established that opiate use dropped from 10.5 percent in September 1971 to 1 percent by early 1973. Among marines in South Vietnam, opiate use peaked at 11.6 percent in December 1972; use declined after urine testing was begun.

Substandard military performance sometimes called attention to drug abuse, but for the most part, minimal standards of performance were maintained. There were drug-dependent soldiers in combat. I visited one medical unit that had been functioning efficiently for some time with a heroin-dependent staff of noncommissioned officers. I also interviewed three soldiers from the combat zone who had fought while having withdrawal symptoms. Their companions vouched for the fact that they had fought. The soldiers said that they had felt wretched. Their efficiency and judgment were no doubt diminished, but under duress, reserves of will and strength enabled them to carry on.

Describing the army's drug users, Robins (1974) indicates that "drug users were disproportionately young, single . . . men from large cities. They tended to have less education, more drug experience before Service, more civilian arrests, and more disciplinary history in Service than men who did not use drugs in Vietnam." Opiate use generally began within six months after arrival in Vietnam, and "there was no correlation between drug use and assignments, danger, or death of friends" (Robins, 1974). Apparently, social pressures and backgrounds were a factor in use. In most of the companies, drug users formed clearly defined, separate groups. Many had constructed clublike retreats where they congregated to use drugs.

Although most soldiers smoked heroin by mixing it with cigarette tobacco, some injected it. Usually, those who injected heroin had also used other methods; users generally did not begin injecting until after they had been smoking for several months. (For those who smoke heroin, injection usually begins when tolerance has been acquired to the limited amount of heroin that can be smoked.) Robins states:

The low rate of injection also depended on the fact that the tour in Vietnam was only one year long for most men. The longer men used heroin, the more likely they were to begin injecting it. Among users who quit within one month, only 7 percent ever injected, but with use between one month and six, the rate increased to 14 percent, with use between six and nine months, to 25 percent, and among those who used more than nine months, the rate of injection rose to 40 percent. Apparently even with very pure heroin, there comes a time when tolerance develops to the point that experiencing euphoria requires injection directly into the vein. [Robins, 1974]

Table 7. *Relation of duration and method of use to persistent heroin use*

Type of heroin use	Soldiers using heroin since leaving Vietnam (%)
Injection before and during tour in Vietnam	73
Injection during tour but not before	26
Smoking only	9

Source: Data from Robins (1974).

Urinalysis at DEROS revealed that 82 percent of those who injected heroin were addicted, compared with only 20 percent of those who smoked (Robins, 1974). The follow-up data also show that there is a relationship between the length of exposure and use of injection and persistent heroin use (Table 7). Robins concludes that heroin injection seems to be the determining factor in persistent heroin use. This is plausible, but there is another interpretation of the data. It is not likely that injection alone could have caused so many heroin users to become addicted, since many more had tried injecting a few times without developing a dependency. What is significant is that those soldiers who injected heroin before and during their tour accounted for most of the persistent addicts; these users had been exposed to heroin use at least ten times longer than the average. Although people do get hooked on the process of injection, duration of use and strength of dose are probably more often the determining factors. Those who reach the point of injecting generally have been using heroin longer than those who smoke it.

Medical personnel in Vietnam felt that withdrawal symptoms for heroin-smoking soldiers were less severe than they would have expected. The same observations were made on those detoxified at regular drug treatment centers in the United States. This may be explained in part by the fact that those who smoked heroin had been exposed to it for a short time. Such evaluations are difficult, however, because the severity of withdrawal depends on many factors and is always subjectively judged.

Use of alcohol and marijuana

Although most soldiers used opiates for the first time in Vietnam and although opiates caused the greatest concern, the use of all drugs increased. The most commonly used drug, with the exception of alcohol, was marijuana. About 41 percent of the soldiers used marijuana before and during their tours of duty in Vietnam. An additional 28 percent began using it there for the first time. Thus, a total of 69 percent of the enlisted men used marijuana.

Not only did the number of soldiers using marijuana rise rapidly, but the frequency of use was higher, and the potency of the drug was five to ten times greater than in the United States. It was common knowledge even among non-users that the marijuana in Vietnam was much stronger. In fact, in both Germany and Vietnam, where potent cannabis was readily available, soldiers escalated rapidly to incredibly high doses of THC in a short time. It was not uncommon for soldiers in Germany to increase their use from one or two stateside marijuana joints a week to 25 or 50 grams of hashish (equal to approximately 100 to 200 marijuana intoxications) a week within three months (Tennant, in U.S. Senate Hearings, 1974). I found no evidence of hashish use among soldiers in Vietnam. This is because the Vietnam marijuana was 10 to 14 percent THC, an even greater potency than Turkish hashish (10 percent THC).

I interviewed several veterans who, upon their return to the United States, were greatly frustrated by the fact that they had become so tolerant to the stronger variety in Vietnam that they were unresponsive to the weaker marijuana available at home.

Although marijuana was not legal in the army and there was some warning against its use, military life offered no real deterrent. Most soldiers (70 percent) reported that marijuana was always available in their companies, and 92 percent reported that it was usually or always available (Robins, 1974). Since each company handled the problem in its own way, there was great variation in attitudes and discipline. Some men complained to me that their captains hassled them for using marijuana (though this was the exception to the rule). The most common attitude was that alcohol and marijuana were problems of about the same magnitude. The long-standing tolerance of alcohol abuse by the armed forces tended to obscure the special problem of marijuana abuse. Alcohol has always been a problem in the army, and the penalties for being drunk on duty are severe. However, drunkenness seems to be kept under fair control, at least to the extent that the efficiency of the men is not threatened. The effects of excessive drinking are difficult to hide and can be dealt with immediately; taking pills or smoking marijuana- or heroin-laced cigarettes can be reasonably unobtrusive. Since 99 percent of the newly enlisted men already used alcohol (Ream, 1972, unpublished data), the number of users did not increase in the service. In fact, it declined to 92 percent, probably because other drugs were so readily available.

Even if there had been no question of the seriousness of the marijuana problem, military authorities would have been cautious about initiating an all-out effort to stop its use. Military leaders could not have stopped the use of marijuana in the army since more and more of the men enlisting were already established users. In fact, excluding marijuana users from enlistment would have amounted to advertising drug abuse as a means for avoiding military service. Had military leaders tried to suppress marijuana use without also starting rehabilitation programs, they would have seen marijuana users switch to alcohol or even heroin. Men regularly using either alcohol or marijuana are agitated if these are not available, and thwarted marijuana users may become aggressive (Kolansky & Moore, 1972*b*).

The army was not prepared to undertake the kind of massive, lengthy rehabilitation programs for heavy users of marijuana that it had for heroin addicts. There was no apparent urgency to deal with marijuana abuse as there had been with heroin. Repressive measures adopted against heroin presented no threats to the military leaders because almost all agreed that heroin was a real problem for both the individual soldier and the military as a whole. It was also easy to test for opiate use, but there was no quick test for marijuana.

I do not imply that inadequate attention was given to the marijuana problem in Vietnam. A special task force of drug abuse specialists developed educational programs that included all the sensual drugs. In the period under study, however, those attempting to present convincing evidence against the use of marijuana were frustrated by the lack of accurate reference works on the subject. It was my own experience that information about drug abuse was well received, but established patterns and attitudes were difficult to break when a soldier had been exposed to discussion sessions for only an hour now and then during his year of duty.

Present information about the effects of marijuana is much more convincing than that available in 1970–1972. It may soon be possible for military leaders to curtail the use of marijuana through education, if young people become less interested in the drug culture as a way of life. Easy tests for marijuana residues may also be developed. The experience of the army in reducing the epidemic of heroin by means of urine tests indicates their effectiveness.

Use of multiple drugs

I have thus far dealt with heroin, marijuana, and alcohol separately because they were handled by the military in different ways. In reality, however, drug users were not generally involved with one drug alone, but with a combination of drugs. Multiple drug use was common before, during, and after a tour of duty in Vietnam. Statistically, it was most likely that a soldier who already used marijuana and/or alcohol heavily would also begin to use heroin for the first time in Vietnam; many drug users tried all three. A soldier rarely gave up a drug when he began to use another. However, a small fraction (11 percent) of the heavy drinkers did not take up heroin in Vietnam, and those who became alcoholics tended to limit their drug use to alcohol.

Amphetamines and barbiturates were each used by about one-fourth of the men in Vietnam. The abuse of these drugs received very little publicity because most of these soldiers also used heroin. Users of multiple drugs tended to use heroin more heavily. Of the narcotics users who also used amphetamines and barbiturates, 60 percent were addicted to narcotics at DEROS; of the narcotics users who did not use amphetamines or barbiturates, 13 percent were addicted (Robins, 1974).

Practical findings from the army experience

Studies of drug abuse in the military have brought to light some important features of addiction and rehabilitation. Cheap, available, potent drugs; powerful peer pressures; and the limited tour of duty combined to make the drug abuse problem in Vietnam unique. There has been no other time when the effects of a drug-using environment could be so clearly seen; young men left their homes, were moved to where drugs were easy to use, and then after about a year returned home. It is not surprising, under these conditions, that drug use rose rapidly in Vietnam.

It is significant that in the ten months of the follow-up study, one-third of the marijuana users and two-thirds of the narcotics users had stopped using their drugs. Going home meant a change in life style and a break from the pattern of drug use that had conditioned them in Vietnam. They adopted the life styles of their social circles. The readjustment was relatively easy because detoxification and withdrawal along with education had largely blunted the driving edge of the addiction process.

In the past, all heroin users who showed withdrawal symptoms were classified as addicts, and it was assumed that all had an equal prospect for rehabilitation. The army data, however, show a clear distinction between users and addicts and between those heavily and lightly addicted. It was estimated that 59 percent of the heroin users had not used heroin regularly enough during the twelve months' stay in Vietnam to have withdrawal symptoms. The other 41 percent used heroin regularly, and most of them were addicted to some extent. For the most part, exposure to opiates was intermittent or brief, and relatively few soldiers developed permanent addiction.

My own sampling of 500 young addicts in the United States showed that many were not able to rehabilitate themselves after a short-term detoxification or a move to a different environment. They tended to remain addicted even if the drug was more expensive or more difficult to obtain. The detoxified soldiers, on the other hand, tended to abstain when they returned home, where potent drugs were used less, more expensive, and less available.

Follow-up data on the group of soldiers in the Robins report ten months after they had left Vietnam show that only 1 percent of all the enlisted men (2.3 percent of those who had used opiates in Vietnam) had permanent addictions. Most of the soldiers in this 1 percent had turned themselves in at DEROS because they were unable to end their narcotic use without help. Although they were detoxified, one in seven (14 percent) remained addicted. These soldiers had used opiates for the longest period of time, and they tended to use multiple drugs.

The length of time heroin is used regularly has a great deal to do with the success of the rehabilitation. Most of the heroin users in Vietnam only started to use heroin there. If addicted at all, they were only addicted for a short time, since the tour of duty was on the average about one year. Those who became readdicted after their return to the United States were mainly those who had used heroin regularly in Vietnam for six months or who had used opiates before going to Vietnam and had become fully addicted early in the tour of duty. Addicts detected at DEROS in Vietnam and detoxified were able to return to intermittent use of heroin or other opiates without reestablishing dependency. This was the case for 10 percent of the Vietnam veterans. Hopefully this 10 percent will stop using opiates, for occasional use may lead to readdiction, and rehabilitation is much more difficult with each episode of addiction.

The army experience gives an optimistic outlook for the recovery of those who quit using opiates early, when the signs of dependency are just developing. This is particularly important, for at least one-third of all marijuana users experiment with opiates. I estimate that, as of 1976, about 8 million people in the United States have tried opiates and that this number is increasing rapidly. Of these, roughly 1 million have already developed persistent dependencies, and probably about one-half are in the incipient stages of dependency. If the users still in the early stages of addiction can be helped, their chances for complete recovery and for a drug-free life are greatly increased.

CHAPTER 8

Rehabilitation

Drug-induced malfunctions that result in sensory deprivation can usually be corrected; the brain's nerve pathways and control centers are disordered, but they remain intact. Destroyed brain cells cannot, of course, be repaired; but the brain has a great capacity for retraining and "rewiring" itself to compensate for losses.

To restore the mechanisms and controls that regulate sensory activity, the entire body must be brought back to a state of health. To accomplish this, there are three phases the rehabilitating addict must go through: he must decide to end his dependence; he must undergo withdrawal; he must struggle through the long period of physical and psychological rehabilitation.

The decision to quit

The drug user must understand the gravity of his situation and the necessity for ending his dependency; his recognition of these facts must lead to a determination to quit. *Only he can make this decision.*

Drug addicts are often terrified of ending drug use. Will detoxification be unbearably painful? What will their companions say? How will they find new friends if they can no longer use drugs? Can they manage a new life stlye? And are there already permanent effects?

Because of the power of the sensual drugs to condition the mind, because of the fear of facing a life without drugs, and because of persistent drug hunger, the commitment to stay off drugs is virtually impossible to keep without help. Although a few addicts are able to stop simply by making up their minds to do so, they are a small minority. An addict no longer has a perspective on himself; he is unable to see unaided that he has been changed for the worse by his drug experience or to admit that he wants to be rehabilitated. He lies to himself and others, is defensive, and develops elaborate rationalizations. Until he reaches the end of his emotional and physical resources, not even the possibility of death seems to deter a severely addicted drug user. When he is high, death is unreal; when he is low (depressed from withdrawal), death is usually perceived as uncertain and secondary to pain. I have observed that although the addict knows intellectually the high injury and death rate among addicts, he feels invulnerable and refuses to recognize that his life is in jeopardy. It is possible that the full powers of reasoning are suppressed or that the addict is motivated by a death wish. As long as any of these situations continue to exist, the possibility for cure is slim. We are reminded of the laboratory animals who stimulate their pleasure centers until they collapse from exhaustion. Fortunately, the reasoning power of the human brain is more highly developed than that of laboratory animals.

The addict can be jolted into an understanding of his situation, but for this he needs help from another person. It is difficult for a parent or spouse to counsel effectively because such a person is usually too closely involved. An informed third party – counselor, doctor, family friend, or teacher – is more likely to be effective, and there is less chance that the addict will reject his advice.

A drug user is best convinced of the harm of drug use when he can verify the evidence. Self-testing, evaluation by a third party, and observations of other addicts can give him such verification.

For the addict who is able to make an honest appraisal of the changes drugs have caused in his physical and mental condition, a self-evaluation can motivate him to end his drug use. The addict may see that his life style has changed; that he has lost his former motivation and goal orientation; that he has little interest in work, school, or his former activities; and that he is no longer interested in other people and cannot sustain personal relationships. He may be able to see from his poor skin color and condition, his lack of energy, and his persistent cough that his health has declined. He may note an inability to sleep deeply and soundly. He may become aware that he has trouble focusing his eyes and that they have become sensitive to light. He may notice that he has become careless about his appearance; that his gait has changed and his motor coordination is poor; that his hands and fingers tremble. He may be able to acknowledge that his speech and thinking have slowed; that he has difficulty concentrating; that his memory is impaired; and that his senses of taste, touch, and smell are not as acute as they once were. He may be able to admit to himself that his ability to function sexually is impaired; that he has lost interest in sex; and that he no longer has sexual dreams. For further discussion of observable changes in the drug user, see Appendix 5.

I have suggested to more than 2,000 marijuana users that they stop using marijuana for several weeks as an experiment. The results have been striking: 520 users reported that their minds became markedly clearer when they tested the effects of abstinence. Many described it as a "lifting of the fog." Even those who used marijuana only occasionally reported an improvement. None of the 2,000 reported negative results. Of the 520 who reported improvement with abstinence, 450 made the decision to quit.

One physician made videotapes of interviews with his drug-using patients and then played the tapes back so that they could see for themselves how much they had changed. The addicts were shaken when they saw they had not been able to disguise their drug use. Their eyes, their gait, their speech, all projected a very different image from the one they thought they were projecting. As a result, several of the addicts decided to quit.

Videotape equipment is not always readily available, but sometimes the same effects can be obtained if someone who knew the addict before he started to use drugs makes a before-and-after comparison of his behavior and attitudes. If the addict knows the evaluation to be objective, it may help convince him to stop.

There is no greater verification of the evidence of the dangers of drug use than for an addict to see drugs kill a friend. This is the most sobering experience most drug users can have, and yet the heavy drug user may not be able to connect himself to this event.

Many addicts are not ready to quit until they have bottomed out, that is, until they realize total emotional and physical depletion. At this point, the addict is worn down physically and wasted by disease and malnutrition. The harried life he leads in the perpetual pursuit of drugs, the worry about arrest, and the isolation and loneliness he feels leave him in a state of deep depression. Finally, the addict can no longer continue this way of life. Once he has sunk to this state, he is often desperate enough to face the fact that he is vulnerable, that death is real, and that the only alternative to death is rehabilitation.

Some authorities on the treatment of drug users feel that an addict must bottom out before he can be helped. They have probably drawn this conclusion from the large number of addicts who leave the rehabilitation centers before they have much hope of being able to stay off drugs. The truth is that many addicts go through withdrawal without any intention of completing the rehabilitation program. Some take the cure merely to lower their tolerance to a cheaper, more manageable level, or so that they can once again get a kick from the drug. Others do it to appease parents, a spouse, or the law. Thus, the high failure rate is a reflection of the large number of addicts who have no commitment to rehabilitation at all rather than of the number whose commitments are weak because they have not yet bottomed out.

The addict does not necessarily have to bottom out, but he must make a firm resolution to quit. Although many addicts have no incentive to quit until they feel near death, I have found that drug users and addicts can be persuaded to undergo rehabilitation before they have bottomed out if they have some powerful incentive. The possibility of recovering their sexual functioning is the kind of incentive that encourages many to make a firm commitment.

First, however, the addict must recognize his sexual and emotional impotence. Nearly all the heroin users I interviewed had failed to face their sexual incapacitation. When drug use became the sole source of sensual pleasure, they ignored or were unaware of their lack of sexual functioning. Once these drug users, many of them young adults in the early stages of addiction, recognized their problem and learned the facts about restoring their sexual capacity, many were persuaded to begin rehabilitation.

Sexual functioning or the lack of it is definite and measurable, and it is vitally important to most people. It may be the eye opener an addict needs to recognize the disorders of his other sensory functions. Just this incentive is enough because all the sensory functions are rehabilitated at the same time by the same process.

It should be stated again here, however, that holding out

the hope of return of sexual and other sensory functioning is just one way of persuading an addict to begin rehabilitation. I have found it to be particularly effective in motivating "new" addicts who are not emotionally disordered (see Appendix 6 for some suggestions). However, the method to be employed depends entirely on how susceptible the addict is to reason, reeducation, and counseling. Those with more severe psychological problems will need more specialized, intensive therapy.

Detoxification

An addict can be forced into detoxification, but his rehabilitation is likely to be more successful and his detoxification easier if he makes the decision to detoxify for himself. Many detoxification centers are secured, however; even though an addict has decided to quit, he may be overcome by the immediate distress of withdrawal and be unable to keep his commitment.

Detoxification from mild drugs can be done at home with the aid of a friend. An addict of hard drugs should always seek professional advice, because detoxification from certain drugs can be dangerous unless it is done under medical supervision. Any large city has many public and private detoxification centers.

Although detoxification is difficult and may even be life-threatening, as long as the addict has the proper care, withdrawal is never so dangerous or painful that he should be deterred from attempting it. Much of the pain is due to fear, which, in fact, intensifies withdrawal symptoms. This is exemplified by the heroin addict who has mild withdrawal symptoms when voluntarily repeating detoxification. He knows what to expect and does not intend to face a life without drugs. Thus, his anxiety is reduced. An addict who is serious about rehabilitation will find detoxification easier if he is educated about the procedure and knows what to expect. The detoxification center should discuss these with the addict before and during withdrawal.

The symptoms of withdrawal are generally the reverse of a drug's acute effects; they range from mild to violent, depending on the drug, the degree of addiction, and the individual.

Marijuana

In detoxification from marijuana, euphoric sensations of the drug high are replaced by irritability and depression; a voracious appetite dwindles; and constant drowsiness is replaced by insomnia. If the use of marijuana is discontinued after two weeks of heavy use, the decline in THC levels on abstinence is marked enough to cause pronounced withdrawal symptoms. The symptoms are not particularly debilitating because there is residual THC and it is released from the system very slowly. Marijuana detoxification, therefore, is no real problem. The user can kick his habit easily and by himself *if he chooses*. The only real difficulty is a psychological one. The user knows that his malaise can be alleviated by another joint, and he can easily become dependent on marijuana again. Recognition of the dangers of marijuana use is often an important deterrent.

Amphetamines and cocaine

The hyperactivity or agitation, the loss of appetite, and the sleeplessness of intoxication give way during abstinence to their opposites: lethargy, sleepiness, a voracious appetite, and depression. During withdrawal, the stimulant user usually eats a great deal and then falls into a deep sleep. His withdrawal is gradual, extending over several days, and accompanied by such symptoms as uneasiness, twitching of the limbs, and perspiration. His determination to live without his drug habit is made extremely difficult by the severe depression that follows his break with the drug. Amphetamine and cocaine users who are only mildly addicted can usually detoxify themselves. But because this depression almost inevitably occurs, and because it sometimes gives rise to thoughts of suicide, detoxifying amphetamine and cocaine users should be given attention for several weeks. Those heavily addicted need medical supervision because they may have more severe withdrawal symptoms, such as hallucinations, heart palpitations, vomiting, diarrhea, and even unconsciousness.

Hallucinogens

Detoxification from the powerful hallucinogens can usually be done in a day, for users rarely build up much tolerance. Sometimes, however, it is necessary to bring someone down from a particularly bad trip. This is usually done with Thorazine (chlorpromazine), a drug that reduces the acute agitation caused by the hallucinogenic effects of LSD. The hallucinogens leave persistent problems: altered personalities, preoccupation, flashbacks, and memory difficulties. These are not remedied by Thorazine or other drugs, and it is not known whether these persisting symptoms are toxic effects or the result of distressing mental experiences.

The user of hallucinogens may have no idea what he is taking. "Mescaline" may really be LSD; or "LSD" may be STP (2,5-dimethyl-4-methylamphetamine, originally synthesized as a motor oil additive, but which has properties somewhat related to those of LSD, mescaline, and the amphetamines). STP is a highly dangerous drug, mainly because it is so often sold as LSD. The difference between the two drugs is critical. Whereas Thorazine counteracts the effects of LSD, it intensifies the effects of STP and can even cause sudden death from cardiovascular collapse. A physician must exercise extreme caution in his treatment when he is not certain what drug an addict has taken.

Heroin

Heroin withdrawal symptoms are distinct. Although they are distressing, they are not at all dangerous. The first signs that opiate withdrawal is beginning are a runny nose and sneezing. Shortly afterward, the skin and the genitals of the addict begin to itch frantically, and no amount of scratching brings relief. A chill then develops; the skin becomes alternately sweaty and clammy; the joints begin to ache; and the flesh becomes painful to the touch. Nausea, vomiting, and uncontrollable defecation (or else extreme constipation) also frequently occur. Throughout, the patient is usually fatigued, hungry, and thirsty, but is unable to eat, drink, or sleep. These symptoms are extremely painful for the first three days. After this, the symptoms begin to fade rapidly, and usually by the eighth day, the addict falls into a short, deep sleep. When he awakens, he is chemically detoxified and suffers no further withdrawal symptoms. For several months after detoxification, however, the addict cannot sleep well and his appetite is depressed. He does not feel well. He has urinary hesitancy. He has difficulty retaining recent information and is unresponsive to other people.

There are several ways a junkie can go about kicking his heroin habit. Surprisingly enough, the easiest and most effective method is for the addict to withdraw cold turkey, that is, simply stop taking the drug and force himself to endure the abstinence syndrome. Heroin withdrawal symptoms are not life-threatening, nor is medical supervision necessary. The week of detoxification, however, is long and agonizing, so reassuring support is an important factor in reducing the risk of relapse. Attempts at self-treatment in isolation only intensify the anxiety the addict feels and increase his difficulty; few people are able to get themselves through withdrawal without yielding to the temptation to relieve their distress by taking the drug again.

A more tedious method of eliminating the drug from the system is for the addict to take decreasing amounts of heroin over an extended period. With this method, detoxification is gradual and the withdrawal symptoms are milder. The disadvantage is that the prolonged period of low-key discomfort is subtly depressing and increases the risk that the addict will return to his habit before withdrawal is complete. Another method is to transfer the addict from intravenously taken heroin to orally administered methadone, a synthetic opiate. Even though the addict no longer uses heroin, he is not actually detoxified, for unless he undergoes withdrawal from methadone, he is as physically dependent on it as he was on heroin. Some addicts can detoxify, however, by first transferring from heroin to methadone and then gradually reducing the dose of methadone. The symptoms of withdrawal from methadone after short use are often milder than those of heroin withdrawal. The dose of methadone can be reduced by 2.5 percent each day without causing definite withdrawal symptoms. Although this method avoids the short-term discomfort of a cold turkey withdrawal, it does not diminish the demoralizing effects of prolonged withdrawal.

Tranquilizing and hypnotic drugs are often used under medical supervision in the treatment of addicts undergoing withdrawal. Librium is commonly used. It reduces pain, anxiety, and the craving for heroin, and promotes sleep. Prolonged use may produce a number of adverse effects, including dependency.

Although the needs of all heroin addicts are not the same, the method I strongly recommend in most cases is the cold turkey withdrawal. The pain is not so severe that it cannot be endured, and if the addict makes a clean break with the drug, he can get through the detoxification quickly. The only real risk is that extreme discomfort will weaken his resolve to rehabilitate. Weakening of resolve occurs less frequently, I have found, after cold turkey withdrawal than when other methods are used, perhaps because a person willing to give up all drugs during detoxification has made a stronger commitment.

Deaddiction centers report that withdrawal symptoms are now milder than they used to be. Some people attribute this to the dilute heroin now being sold on the streets. This is probably a factor, but I have seen moderate withdrawal symptoms in addicts who had been using pure heroin. I attribute the milder symptoms to the fact that as the heroin culture expands, addicts know more about withdrawal and feel less anxiety about it.

Alcohol

Withdrawal for the alcoholic is much more difficult. The abstinence syndrome is not only painful, but can even be fatal. If allowed to develop unchecked, the symptoms are nausea, anxiety, agitation, confusion, tremors, and hallucinations. When particularly severe, the symptoms are called delirium tremens and can cause cardiovascular collapse and death. When given the proper treatment, however, the patient's condition usually improves in a very short time.

Because the withdrawal illness is so severe, the late-stage alcoholic should not try to detoxify himself. He needs medical assistance and may even require hospitalization. The treatment usually involves controlling the withdrawal symptoms through the administration of gradually decreasing doses of medication – commonly Valium or Librium. Cardiac arrest is the biggest risk during the period of acute withdrawal.

Many alcoholics use barbiturates to help counteract withdrawal symptoms. Frequently, they combine alcohol and barbiturates to get an effect that surpasses that of either drug used by itself. This combination is extremely hazardous: the effects are more than additive and can easily result in serious intoxication or death from overdose. Detoxification must be done under medical supervision.

Barbiturates

Barbiturate detoxification is quite similar to alcohol withdrawal, but is even more dangerous. If a barbiturate addict stops taking the drug abruptly, severe symptoms appear. For several hours after the user takes his last dose, while the effects of intoxication are wearing off, the user's condition may appear to improve. Within one and one-half to five days, however, weakness, dizziness, anxiety, tremors, and hyperactivity develop, followed by epileptiform seizures that sometimes result in death. Between the third and seventh days, delusions and hallucinations appear, and there may be uncontrollable hostility and violence. This behavior resembles the symptoms of a severe psychosis. Similar to delirium tremens, the condition may last for days and may not subside for months.

Barbiturate addicts should always be detoxified under medically supervised conditions. Because the withdrawal symptoms should not be allowed to appear, the physician first determines the dose for which the addict has developed a tolerance and then administers that amount. The margin between tolerance and overdose is small, so caution must be used. Gradually, over a period of weeks, the dose is reduced. If any signs of the abstinence syndrome appear, the dose is increased until they disappear, then the gradual withdrawal is begun again. The patient is observed closely, his diet is controlled, and he is usually given additional treatment to counteract the physical disorders caused by his heavy use of the drug.

Minor tranquilizers

Minor tranquilizers are usually used in combination with other sensual drugs. In general, withdrawal from tranquilizers is similar to barbiturate withdrawal and can be just as dangerous. As is true of barbiturate and alcohol addicts, those hooked on tranquilizers should always be detoxified under medical supervision.

Physical and psychological rehabilitation

With proper care, the addict can usually overcome chemical dependence without too much difficulty. This is only the beginning of a long road to recovery. The addict's body and mind have both been severely affected and both must be rehabilitated. He must change his way of life and his way of thinking about himself. This may be difficult, but the addict can be helped and, more important, can help himself to make these changes. Some of the elements I feel are part of any successful recovery are discussed below.

Education

Educating the addict about the debilitating effects of drugs on the pleasure mechanisms can give him a strong incentive to rehabilitate himself. The addict becomes an expert on the sensations he gets from taking drugs, but he does not understand what drugs do to his sexual and other pleasure mechanisms.

The drive to seek pleasure and avoid pain can be just as powerful a force in getting an addict to stop drug use as it was in getting him started. The pleasure mechanisms are slow to recover, however, and if the recovery takes too long, the addict may take up drugs again. In such a case, the drive to avoid pain or to feel immediate pleasure is stronger than the attractions of a drug-free future. Keeping an addict off drugs long enough for his pleasure mechanisms to recover is made easier if, during the period of rehabilitation, he is encouraged about the restoration of his sexual and other sensual functioning and if he is able to recognize his progress, even though slow.

A detoxified user sometimes returns to drugs because he is not given enough information or help during the period after detoxification. He still does not feel well, his sexual functions are still depressed, and he is unable to sleep soundly. If he is not informed that this will be the case, he may think these are signs of permanent damage and become discouraged; if he is fully informed about the rehabilitation process, he will be more willing to wait out this difficult period. Because reversing psychological conditioning and recovering sensual functioning take time, the addict's drug hunger may last for months or years. His brain's controls have to adjust to be able to work well again without the drug, and he has to adjust to a new life style. He must be prepared and willing to wait.

Because the addict's short-term memory and continuity of thought are usually affected by drugs, he may be overwhelmed if he is given too much advice and information. Moreover, his defensive system works to maintain his self-image; recognizing his deteriorated state and accepting advice may be too threatening to him. He may deny what is said to him and be unable to take in information. Therefore, material must be presented in a positive and objective manner. Because the addict is likely to be able to absorb only what he needs at the moment, information may have to be repeated to him over and over.

Drug-free environment

The detoxified addict must be kept away from other drug users until he can develop sufficient stamina to stay "clean." He should not live at home immediately after detoxification if he lives close to former drug contacts and drug-using friends; his inner struggle to abstain will be difficult enough without additional temptations and pressures.

The detoxified addict should be prepared for drug hunger, which will stay with him for a long time. Drug hunger seems to come on in cycles and is as strong as the normal desire for sex.

Some detoxified addicts are able to keep the commitments they make themselves; others cannot remain drug-free longer than the time it takes to contact their suppliers after they leave the detoxification center. In one study of fifty heroin addicts who voluntarily entered a treatment clinic, over half, after withdrawal from heroin, left the hospital against medical advice to take drugs again to relieve unbearable feelings (Chessick, 1960).

Often, the former drug user who feels he has fully recovered and has overcome his dependency believes he can use drugs again occasionally without becoming addicted. He remembers his initial experience with the drug when the effects were keen and uncomplicated by dependency. What the long-term addict does not understand and what drug experts are at a loss to explain, is that he usually cannot take the drug again, even once, without returning to full dependency. There are residual effects from his former state of dependency that produce drug hunger and susceptibility, but it is not known whether this is a psychological or a physiological phenomenon. All we know is that drugs pose a threat to the ex-addict for the rest of his life. Alcoholics Anonymous says that there is no such thing as an ex-alcoholic, and so it is with other addictive sensual drugs.

Even former cigarette smokers find that if they start smoking again, they are soon smoking as many cigarettes as they did when they stopped.

Detoxifying addicts may substitute one drug for another, and users of multiple drugs may try to eliminate only one habit. Those who quit using narcotics often begin to use cigarettes, alcohol, or marijuana heavily. For the most rapid and complete cure, the addict should refrain from the use of all sensual drugs. It is very significant that, in my sampling of college males, those who used illegal drugs were more likely to be drinkers or heavy smokers than those who did not. Many rehabilitation centers require abstinence from all drugs, including tobacco and alcohol – a practice I strongly endorse.

There is no safe drug. No sensual drug can substitute for the body's own resources and capacities for pleasure.

Family support and counseling

The support of the addict's family is, of course, a great help; without it, rehabilitation can be more difficult. The family, however, cannot always give the kind of help an addict needs. The members of the family may be too emotionally involved; they may have contributed in some way to the addiction; or they may lack the time and energy needed to help. The addict may feel uncomfortable with them because of their expectations and judgments.

The members of the family may not be prepared to handle the rehabilitating addict's problems, but he needs their constant love and moral support. These may be hard to give to an unappreciative and hostile addict, but there is nothing he needs more. I have found addicts to be desperately lonely people; although they put on a brave front, they crave love and a feeling of belonging.

This does not imply that the addict should be pampered,

overprotected, and indulged. An addict must somehow be made to realize that he is responsible for his drug use. Parents do a child a great disservice if they allow him to hide behind excuses. Parents too often minimize their child's drug use to defend their own use of tobacco or alcohol, to avoid coping with the problem, or to show they still accept the child. Some of the most common excuses are "the school is full of drug users"; or "after all, adults use pills and alcohol"; or "the problems for youth are so great, it's little wonder they resort to drugs"; or "it isn't his fault – he was seduced into drug use." Valid or not, such dodges do not help the drug user. If parents do not take a stand against drug use, the child cannot be expected to. A child is often relieved to have his drug use stopped by the law or his parents; he needs firmness, not excuses.

Often those closest to the addict are unaware of what is involved in rehabilitation and what their role should be. In many cities programs are available to help families understand the problems of the former drug user and gain insight into what caused him to take drugs. While family members may not be the most effective counselors for the addict, they can provide special assurance in their support of his rehabilitation program, in their efforts to understand the problem, and in their genuine concern for him.

The most effective help usually comes from a third-party counselor, one who is trained and thoroughly understands the problems of addiction. It is often the relationship that develops between the addict and his counselor that is crucial.

During his addiction, the addict has regressed to an earlier state of emotional development. He is egocentric; he wants immediate gratification; he lacks ability to take responsibility; and he attempts to gratify his needs in antisocial ways. While he was an addict, the drug was the sole source of his needs and gratification. The counselor will help him discover and define what his needs without drugs are and help him explore alternative ways of fulfilling them. The addict may have serious doubts about his own worth and abilities. The counselor can help him regain his self-respect and confidence.

The addict must also develop social awareness. If he can develop positive feelings toward himself and regain a sense of his own worth, he can learn to understand the needs of others and will be able to develop successful social relationships. The counselor can help him accomplish all these goals.

Techniques and approaches vary from counselor to counselor, and the addict may have to search for one he can have rapport with and who can help him meet his particular needs. I have observed that drug addicts make the most progress when the counselor is somewhat authoritative and firm in setting limits. This approach, of course, must be balanced with sympathy and understanding. The counselor must also adjust his treatment to the addict's health, the degree of brain damage, his psychological problems, and his legal, environmental, and economic situation.

The addict will undoubtedly test the limits set by the counselor, who must be alert to the addict's deceptions. The counselor must not let the addict fool himself into believing that a meeting with an old friend will not hurt, that he is not an addict, that one more dose is all right, or that he can get by without help.

The counselor may ask the addict to set some goals. These may be as simple and direct as cleaning his room or eating three meals every day. Whatever the goals, they must be consistent and must demand regularity and persistence from the addict; and they must be attainable, because the addict needs success. His capability will be limited at first, but as he finds himself able to handle limited goals, he will gradually be able to deal with bigger and bigger problems. The counselor can help the addict take one day at a time and learn to assess his progress.

Food, rest, and medical attention

The internal body rhythms are usually acutely disturbed both by the drugs and by the life that dependency forces the addict to lead. The addict does not get hungry and does not eat well; he sleeps little or sporadically and lightly; and he gets almost no exercise. His life style has made him susceptible to infections and diseases. To rebuild his strength and resistance to infection and to improve his health and emotional outlook, the drug addict should obtain an adequate amount of rest, have adequate medical treatment, and eat a balanced diet.

Early in recovery, a quiet setting with little external stimulation seems most satisfactory. Sleeping conditions are important, since disturbed sleep may continue for months after detoxification. In military rehabilitation centers, patients who were moved from large wards with double bunks to single beds with not more than six persons to a room slept better and recovered more quickly. Even more privacy is desirable. Undisturbed sleep is important for many reasons. One researcher reports that growth hormone secretion can actually be prevented by waking a subject periodically during the night each time he appears to be going into a deep sleep. If, after five or six hours of being repeatedly awakened, the subject is allowed to fall into deep sleep, a growth hormone rise then appears (Frohman, 1975).

Food, too, is important. Food is more than the vitamins, minerals, and calories it provides; it is said that "a good meal, appetizingly set forth, satisfies not only the body but also something in the soul." Food and shelter are often symbols of security to the addict who, ever since he became hooked, has rarely had constant means of support. Eventually, he must establish a regular eating and sleeping routine in order to restore the normal tempo of his bodily rhythms.

Exercise

Regular exercise is almost as important as a drug-free environment for the rehabilitating addict. Physical exertion actually expands the mental and physical powers, helps restore the body's cyclic rhythms, and accelerates the whole recovery process. Exercise not only increases general body activity, but it also, as we now know, increases brain activity.

More vigorous exercise should be required of the rehabilitating addict than most programs offer. Under normal circumstances, it usually takes a young person six to eight weeks of workouts to achieve good physical conditioning. It takes the former addict somewhat longer, depending on his level of debilitation. In general, however, the heavier the exercise or work load (adjusted for individual capacity), the more rapid and complete the recovery.

The ex-addict's sexual capacities are also restored more quickly through exercise. The feeling of health gained through physical exertion is closely linked to sexual performance. In addition, exercise also seems to increase the production of semen, which fills the seminal organs and enhances the desire for sexual activity.

Natural stimulation of the pleasure centers

As rehabilitation progresses, a former drug user should be given more and more opportunities to stimulate his pleasure centers naturally. As far as we know, only in the human brain can thinking activate the pleasure mechanism; in man the limbic pleasure centers can be activated not only by the sense organs but also by the thinking regions of the brain. We can learn to relax muscles, be more aware of sights, sounds, smells, tastes, and touch, and increase our sexual pleasures. The brain has a storehouse of treasures that only need to be remembered and associated with present and past activities.

The rehabilitating addict should be encouraged to engage in activities that require thinking, communicating, reading, and studying. He needs to relearn an awareness of the world and become sensitive to natural sources of pleasure.

Spiritual power

Many hard drug addicts have been able to withdraw for a time from a drug, but unless they find positive alternatives to take the place of the drug, they lapse into a cycle of use, withdrawal, and reuse. Among the heroin addicts I have helped, those most successful at breaking the use-withdrawal cycle were the ones who turned to a spiritual power for help. Alcoholics Anonymous has found this principle fundamental to the success of their program, and addicts who have sought help through organized religion have profited consistently. AA does not encourage creed or ritual, but believes that since the alcoholic has not been able to manage things himself, he will be better off if he turns his life over to the care of a power greater than himself. The Salvation Army has been successful in helping addicts, and the National Council for the Prevention of Drug Abuse also emphasizes Christianity in helping the addict through his rehabilitation.

Why an addict should still be capable of deep religious feelings when all other sensations and experiences have vanished cannot be fully explained. From my interviews with addicts, however, I have discovered that the capacity for religious response remains in spite of drug-induced sensory deprivation. Once spiritual insight has been felt, it helps the addict to get off drugs and stay off and to recover his capacity for sensual gratification.

Twenty-seven male and one female addicts have told me independently about remarkable religious experiences that helped them end severe drug addictions. As drug addicts, they had reached the bottom. They were emaciated, severely ill, no longer responsive to intravenous heroin or amphetamines, sensually and sexually impotent, and paranoid. They also had premonitions of death. Although most of them had not been religious, they decided to pray, either out of desperation or in preparation for death. They asked to be cured of drug illness and dependency; and, while praying, each had a profound spiritual experience including sensation of bright lights. They slept after they prayed and, on awakening, found their attitudes completely changed. They stopped taking drugs and had only mild or no withdrawal symptoms. All found that their sensual capacities returned quickly.

Even if an addict does not have such a dramatic experience, he can still feel spiritual ecstasy when other sensual feelings have been obliterated by drugs. The mechanism in the brain for experiencing spirituality may be independent of the sensual mechanisms, and perhaps sensual gratifications can be reactivated by the powerful stimulation of a spiritual insight.

The addict needs support in his struggle to give up drugs. Religion can often fill this need. It offers the addict support and strengthens his willpower. I encourage the addict who seeks my advice to consider adopting the religion that is natural to his origin and culture and that will give him the most help.

Methods of treatment and rehabilitation programs

Selecting a rehabilitation program is not easy; each addict has individual problems and needs, and the rehabilitation programs are limited. Even though thousands of treatment centers have been established in cities all over the country, there are not enough trained personnel or facilities to rehabilitate the increasing number of addicts properly. Additionally, publicly financed rehabilitation programs are difficult to administer. Most public centers are pressed to admit too many for treatment because of the otherwise prohibitive costs; yet for his recovery, the addict needs extensive, individual attention and professional counseling. Good programs are available, however, both publicly and privately financed.

Since opinions on treatment methods vary even among the experts, each program must be evaluated for its merits in relation to the addict. Someone who knows the addict well should assess his situation carefully and help him choose a proper method of rehabilitation. It is important that the addict agree to the choice. If possible, before a commitment is made, a program should be observed. Although each program has something to offer, no matter how good it appears on paper, its personnel are the backbone. Programs vary. Some are loosely knit; others are highly organized; some require living in; others are drop-in centers. Some centers reach out to addicts in jails, hospitals, and on the streets. Some are only for detoxification, while others take drug users only after they are detoxified; some do both. Many private industries offer clinics to help employees with drug problems.

To get information about drug treatment centers in your area, contact the following local, state, or federal sources. If they cannot supply you with the information you are seeking, they can direct you to a source:

Libraries (books are available
  on drug abuse programs)
Mental health association
Public mental health clinics
Hospitals

Private physician
Nurses' association
Red Cross association
Police department
Schools
Religious centers
City information services
Health department
Medical association

The failure rate at most centers for drug treatment is high, probably much higher than most centers will admit. Follow-up studies are difficult to conduct, and many programs consider in their figures only those addicts who have been in the program for at least three months. Addicts often enter a center without a firm commitment. They are compelled to do so by court orders or by their families, or they agree to detoxification only to reduce their tolerance for the drug or because they have become dangerously ill. They fall back into their old habits when they leave the center. The success or failure of a program depends on the motivation of the addict himself.

The therapeutic and encounter methods of treatment, rap sessions, testimonials, and prayers are some of the approaches used in rehabilitation programs. Most programs, in order to reach as many addicts as possible, use a combination of approaches. Some of the common characteristics of the therapeutic and the encounter methods are described here.

Therapeutic treatment

Therapeutic treatment is the name given to a method of live-in treatment in which the treatment center plays the role of an extended family with a strong, autocratic leader who rules the house. Strict demands are placed upon the addict's behavior, and in many ways, he is treated like a child. This can be valuable since, like a child, an addict has lost his sense of responsibility and his perception of long-range goals. This method of treatment assumes that an addict's drug problem is symptomatic of other emotional and social problems; that the addict has lost his personal and social bearings; and that once he has been helped to deal with these underlying problems, he can recover.

After an addict has been admitted to this type of treatment center, he begins at the bottom of the job ladder with, perhaps, latrine duty or dishwashing. As he proves himself worthy of trust and responsibility, he moves up to more desirable jobs. Often room assignments are made according to the same standard: the addict is first given the smallest, darkest room and, if he merits it, is then advanced to lighter, more pleasant surroundings. The rules of the house are usually strict, and infraction results in demotion and disapproval. In this way, the addict learns to see his behavior in social terms. He begins to make a connection between his own actions and the welfare of the group, begins to see the necessity for self-control and responsibility, and develops a sense of involvement with the goals of the social microcosm. Sanctions or disapproval for his behavior come from both the leader of the house and other residents. They are allowed to tell the addict what he is doing wrong, how his behavior is offensive, and how his attitude may endanger the welfare of the members of the house. He is thus given a moral model to emulate and the weight of social approval to enforce his adjustment to it.

Encounter therapy

Both live-in and drop-in rehabilitation centers may use encounter therapy in their rehabilitation programs. Small groups meet several times a week to discuss, analyze, and confront one another. Here, each addict can let off steam and tell other members of the group what is bothering him. Anything but physical violence is allowed, and the only demand is for honesty.

This kind of therapy is meant to force the addict to confront the sources of his hostility and isolation from other people. It makes him see himself as others see him and prevents him from hiding behind a facade; he is forced to see through his rationalizations for drug use and to interact with others who do not use drugs. The confrontations are often brutal, since the object of the encounter is to bring into the open the most sensitive areas of feeling.

Each group has a leader who directs the session and prevents it from turning into a free-for-all. He guides the group so that the encounter is helpful and constructive to the members. He is responsible for controlling and working through a confrontation to a positive resolution.

In my opinion, encounter therapy, unless carefully controlled and directed, is dangerous. It has proved damaging to some personalities, especially the young. There is nothing so brutal for a teenager as an attack from his peers. For someone who can respond to the encounter group technique, however, the peer pressure it relies on can be a powerful influence.

Rehabilitation programs in the United States

The methods of four of the larger, better known American organizations and one of the small outpatient programs are presented here as examples of the various kinds of treatment available. The large organizations do not necessarily have better programs than smaller or less well-known organizations, but they typify the approaches.

Alcoholics Anonymous. One of the most successful groups in treating the problems of alcoholics, AA began in the

1930s and is now a worldwide organization of 14,000 loosely organized groups. The only requirement for membership is a desire to stop drinking; AA has no dues or fees and is supported through contributions of its members; it does not keep membership records; it is not allied with any organization or institution; it does not wish to engage in controversy. Its only purpose is to help alcoholics stay sober. AA does not claim to cure the alcoholic, but to control his illness; its philosophy is that no alcoholic can ever return even to moderate social drinking. AA members meet with each other to relate experiences and ideas, but the basis of the rehabilitation program is the Twelve Steps toward rehabilitation:

1. We admit we were powerless over alcohol – that our lives had become unmanageable.

2. We came to believe that a Power greater than ourselves could restore us to sanity.

3. We made a decision to turn our will and our lives over to the care of God *as we understand Him*.

4. We made a searching and fearless moral inventory of ourselves.

5. We admitted to God, to ourselves, and to another human being the exact nature of our wrongs.

6. We were entirely ready to have God remove all these defects of character.

7. We humbly asked Him to remove our shortcomings.

8. We made a list of all persons we had harmed and became willing to make amends to them all.

9. We made direct amends to such people wherever possible except when to do so would injure them or others.

10. We continued to take personal inventory and when we were wrong promptly admitted it.

11. We sought through prayer and meditation to improve our conscious contact with God *as we understand Him*, praying only for knowledge of His will and the power to carry out that will.

12. Having had a spiritual awakening as the result of these steps, we tried to carry this message to alcoholics and to practice these principles in all our affairs.

Although AA is spiritually based, it is not a religious movement. Wherever the word God appears in its program, AA translates it to mean a greater power "as you understand Him." This has enabled the AA program to help people from all faiths, as well as nonreligious people.

With the recent, rapid increase in alcoholism among youth, new groups are being formed in the larger cities, under the sponsorship of AA, called Young People's AA (YPAA). Cooperating with the AA are groups for families of alcoholics (Al-Anon) and for teenage children of alcoholics (Alateen).

In general, the problems of the alcoholic are the same as those of other drug addicts, and many of the live-in and drop-in programs pattern some of their methods after those of AA. For example, all the programs I am familiar with recognize that an addict cannot be helped until he accepts that he is an addict and wants to be helped; most use ex-addicts in their recovery programs; and all believe that a power greater than the individual (this power may even be the group) can help the addict get off drugs. Narcotics Anonymous, which started in 1953, is such a group. It utilizes nonprofessional group therapy and AA's steps to recovery. Like AA, Narcotics Anonymous holds that there are no ex-addicts, only addicts who do not and must not take drugs.

After a former drug user has left a live-in rehabilitation center, he needs all the support he can get from his friends and family. He may find it helpful to become a member of one of the many organizations for ex-addicts.

Synanon. Synanon, the first therapeutic community for drug addicts, began in 1958 in California with a small group of drug users. Today, it houses nearly 1,500 people, mostly ex-addicts, in its various centers. The salient features of the Synanon movement are the self-imposed poverty of the members and their willingness to place their future in the hands of the organization. Therapeutic treatment and encounter therapy are used to break the addict of old habits and to encourage participation in the life of the Synanon community.

Synanon is a self-contained community and discourages reentry into society. It gives its members jobs within the organization, a place to live, and a miniature social structure. About one-third of those who enter Synanon leave treatment within thirty days. These people may feel an aversion to encounter therapy and resent the harsh initial treatment; they may find it impossible to make a commitment to live and work at Synanon because of family or jobs; or they may simply be unable to conform to the Synanon life style. For those who choose to stay, however, Synanon offers a way of life free from drugs.

Phoenix House. Begun in New York in 1967, Phoenix House has grown from a group of five ex-addicts determined to stay free of drugs to an organization of twenty-one centers with about ninety people in each. Phoenix House uses both therapeutic and encounter treatment, but unlike Synanon, its goal is to return the ex-addict to society. During the addict's stay, between eighteen months and two years, every effort is made to prepare him for reentry into the community. Job-training programs are offered, and formal education classes are given at the center by the New York public school system. When a resident is almost ready to leave the house, he may leave each day to work, attend school, or get special job training. To help with a family situation, the parents or spouse of the addict are encouraged to attend special weekly encounter sessions.

Teen Challenge. This program, begun in 1958 in New York, was founded by David Wilkerson, an Assemblies of God minister. There are now about forty centers located in major cities throughout the United States, Canada, and Europe. Teen Challenge is a specifically therapeutic community with both live-in and drop-in centers. The leaders emphasize spiritual redirection and conversion through Christ. They concentrate on rehabilitation of the "whole man" and not simply on his addiction – which, they believe, is only symptomatic of greater problems in the individual. They believe the addict must establish a new basis and new goals for his life that are based on his spiritual understanding.

Teen Challenge admits that it can only help the person who is desperate for help, not the one who just wants to control his habit. It offers a caring community whose goals are to return the addict to his family and to offer a spiritual alternative to the drug culture. The community offers its support to the members in group and individual counseling sessions. It is firmly against attack therapy, believing that the addict is already torn down and needs to rebuild his self-confidence, self-discipline, and social relationships.

The community imposes a strict discipline on a new member until he gives evidence of self-discipline and maturity. The organization offers the addict relief from heavy financial burdens and a chance for trade and vocational training or formal education through the state department of vocational rehabilitation. The program is open to anyone who sincerely feels he needs help and who shows a willingness to be honest about his problem.

Dr. Baird's program. Robert Baird, of New York City, single-handedly runs one of the most successful outpatient programs I have witnessed. By day, he is a practicing physician on Fifth Avenue, New York; at night, he runs a free clinic in a poor neighborhood in upper Manhattan. Addicts who have genuinely decided to quit drug use attend nightly sessions for a year. Baird is an effective group leader: he is a strong father figure; he gives love and kindness, but he is firm and unbending about drug use. He encourages parents, husbands, and wives of addicts to attend the nightly sessions and enlists their cooperation in helping the addict.

Rehabilitation programs in other countries

Some countries have established rehabilitation facilities for their own citizens, but the rise in drug use among the mobile youth from the Western countries has created a need for rehabilitation centers to help these young travelers.

For many reasons – adventure, low living costs, cheap drugs – addicts from the Western world travel the "hashish trail." The route they follow goes through Yugoslavia, Greece, Turkey, and Iran to India and other nearby countries. Labin (U.S. Senate Hearings, Part II, 1972; see Appendix 7), who traveled the hashish trail from Western Europe to Goa studying the drug problem, estimated that only about 25 percent of the young drug users who start get as far as Afghanistan. Most return to their own countries before they get too far. Some, however, get to India, Nepal, and Goa. Labin has described the wretched lives of these young people. At the time of her travels, she estimated that 40 percent of the addicts were American; the rest were English, German, Scandinavian, French, Dutch, Australian, Italian, and Belgian.

I spent an evening in a cheap hotel and restaurant in Kabul patronized by drug addicts from the Western countries. They were thin, lifeless, and obviously in need of a good meal. However, they preferred to spend any money they had for drugs rather than food. They were lonely and lost; their drug use consumed most of their energy and thoughts.

My wife and I visited a third-floor hashish shop in Katmandu. Going up the winding stairs, we passed small drug dens where young drug users were sitting. Those who were not too spaced out looked at us suspiciously as we passed. When it became obvious we were not there to criticize them, several drifted into the tiny shop. They listened to our conversation; a few of the more alert entered into the discussion now and then. When we left, they drifted back to their drug dens.

I have visited rehabilitation centers around the world set up to help young drug users. Most are similar to treatment centers in the United States. The addictions and problems they treat depend on the drugs locally available and used.

I visited an effective army drug rehabilitation center, located in a former private country club in the hills of the German countryside. The atmosphere was rural and peaceful; the ratio of trained personnel to addicts was high. Each addict was to remain in the program for several months. Army discipline was combined with warmth and concern. The center had a vigorous exercise and athletic program and offered classes in mathematics, science, and crafts. Daily chores were assigned, and social programs were organized. The addicts were allowed free time and given excellent food.

There I met privately with soldiers undergoing rehabilitation treatment for heroin dependency. They were very concerned about their lost sexual potency and, as is usually the case in drug rehabilitation programs, had not been counseled about it. They were apathetic about their exercise program until they realized that exercise would speed their recovery.

Another successful rehabilitation center was the Life of the World. For young men, this center was in a seventy-room, 300-year-old mansion in the hills of Gloucestershire, England. Founded in 1967 by Reverend Frank Wilson, the center combined strict rules with love and the Christian faith. Among its special physical features were extensive gardens, fruit orchards, a farm, a printing shop, and a combination meeting hall, theater, and sports arena. Restoration of the old mansion was part of the rehabilitation program. The addicts stayed from six to twelve months and worked eight hours a day, interrupted only by group meetings. They worked in teams on the farm, in the print shop, or in the maintenance and building crew for the main house. Evening activities covered a whole range of interests such as indoor and outdoor sports, music, art, handicrafts, cookery, Bible studies, chapel services, and films.

In Kabul, Afghanistan, I spent a day with a successful live-in rehabilitation group. It was, again, one that used firmness, love, and Christian faith. I was surprised to find such a lively, well-run center in that remote part of the world. A three-story house was filled with young men and women from all parts of the world who had come to Kabul for the drug scene and who had ended up needing help. The house was run by a young, enthusiastic American couple. The addicts had a daily program to follow, which included chores to help run the house. They could leave the program whenever they wished. In Katmandu I visited a similar center that was just being established.

It is clear that no country is exempt from drug abuse, and all are making efforts to deal with the problem. Professor Miras of the University of Athens told me of a unique rehabilitation center he helps administer, located on an Athenian beach, for drug addicts who gather in Athens during the summer.

In populations where there is strong social feeling against drug abuse, where there are close family ties, and where the youth participate in a religion that does not condone drug use, drugs are much less likely to be used. Even in countries where drug use is endemic, it was restricted until recently to a segment of the population. However, with easy transportation and communication, the drug problem is spreading even into those areas where the youthful population was considered drug-free. For example, I was told by the authorities that the Nepalese people, like those of other countries on the drug trail, were becoming worried because their young were being introduced to drug use by foreign travelers.

Maintenance and substitution programs

Drug maintenance programs and opiate substitutions are nothing new. Several times in the past, when opiate addiction grew to epidemic proportions, new opiates were substituted for old ones in efforts to control the spreading addiction.

Morphine, when it was first isolated from opium in 1805, was used in Hong Kong to "cure" opiate addiction. In America during the Civil War, morphine and codeine were injected intravenously with the newly invented hypodermic needle and were used indiscriminately as pain killers. The result was that thousands of injured men contracted the "soldier's disease." The problem was serious; after the war, the number of morphine addicts was estimated at 400,000, or about 12 percent of the population. Work was done to find a new cure, and in 1898 a new drug was synthesized from morphine. Purported to be nonaddictive when used in place of morphine, the new wonder drug was called heroin.

From the time of its synthesis until the early part of this century, restriction on the sale of heroin in the United States was minimal. In addition to those unwittingly addicted by overprescription, many became addicted through the use of cure-all patent medicines that contained opiates. If a legal prescription for medical purposes was not in order, an addict could readily purchase heroin by bribing certain physicians and pharmacists. In 1914, the Harrison Nar-

cotics Act was passed to regulate the production, manufacture, and distribution of narcotics. The first narcotic
dispensing clinic was opened in New York in 1918, and
forty-four such clinics were opened subsequently around
the country. A day's supply of morphine, heroin, or cocaine
was dispensed free, but the dose was gradually reduced in an
attempt to wean the addict from the drug. In five years, all
the clinics were closed; the government had determined
that they contributed to the spread of addiction, the growth
of a black market, and the rise in crime.

The need for a new cure for heroin addiction rose from
the present heroin epidemic. In the early 1960s there were
only about 50,000 opiate addicts. In 1976, estimates of the
number of heroin addicts ranged from 400,000 to 2 million.

Drug maintenance programs are an alternate means of
rehabilitation for the opiate addict. Usually such programs
maintain the addict with enough of the drug to prevent
withdrawal symptoms without producing euphoria. This
dose is just enough to keep in balance the body mechanisms
that have become adjusted to work only with heroin in the
system. Ideally, the addict's doses are decreased until he is
drug-free. Stabilizing doses are difficult to determine, however, and the margin of dose for a given range of effects is
narrow. If too much is given, euphoria is produced (with the
additional possibility of overdose); if too little is given, the
addict may seek additional drugs. For the addict who cannot
function entirely drug-free, a maintenance program has
proved most helpful. The proper stabilizing dose not only
prevents withdrawal symptoms, but also suppresses some
anxiety.

The main difficulty in trying to establish a maintenance
program of any kind is that maintenance doses do not work
for people who are seeking the drug's sensual effects. A
tolerance develops and the dose must then be increased.
Dispensaries cannot control the spread of opiates if they are

already available on the streets; as long as sufficient opiates are available, addicts will increase their doses and perhaps even go through withdrawal voluntarily, to start over at low doses. Middle-aged addicts are often willing to accept maintenance doses, but young adults are more sensually demanding and find it difficult to discipline themselves to a maintenance program.

Methadone substitution: the hope

For years, scientists have been searching for a drug that would prevent withdrawal symptoms, eliminate drug hunger, and block the sensual effects of heroin. They thought methadone was such a drug, and methadone clinics were opened on a large scale in the United States in 1971.

Methadone substitution: the clinics

Methadone clinics in the United States are funded locally or by state or federal government and are controlled by federal regulations. Initially the regulations were lax, causing a methadone black market to develop at an alarming rate. In an attempt to remedy this situation, federal regulations have been tightened. The clinics and physicians are licensed. Approved outlets supply the methadone to the clinics. Patients are required to have been opiate addicts for at least two years before they are admitted. All new patients must drink the methadone at the clinic, and after that a patient may never take home more than a three-day supply. Urine samples are taken once a week. There are detailed regulations covering all aspects of admission, dispensing, security, and record keeping. Regulations vary from state to state, as the states may make laws that are stricter than federal laws.

Methadone substitution: the fallacies

Many of the arguments originally used in support of methadone programs have since been disproved. These arguments are stated below and their fallacy explained.

Methadone is a special drug. After methadone was first used experimentally to treat heroin addiction (by Dole and Nyswander in 1964), it was thought that methadone had all the virtues and none of the drawbacks of opiates. This has since been disproved. Methadone is, in fact, a synthetic opiate with the same fundamental chemical structure as opiates derived from the opium poppy. All opiates related to morphine are essentially interchangeable; the addict can substitute heroin, morphine, Demerol, opium, codeine, or methadone for the drug to which he is addicted. The sensual effects, however, and the doses needed to obtain these effects vary. Methadone more closely approximates morphine than it does heroin. It was, in fact, developed by the Nazis during World War II when their supply of morphine ran low.

The results reported by Dole and Nyswander (1965), which were widely quoted as evidence for the success of the methadone treatment method and which led to the opening of many methadone clinics, were not brought about by the special chemical properties of methadone. The variables in the Methadone Maintenance Treatment Program, as the Dole-Nyswander project was called, were carefully controlled (Epstein, 1974). Volunteers for treatment were screened. More than two-thirds of the addicts selected were over thirty years old; a large number had not recently been criminally active. Having been on a waiting list for six months to a year before being accepted into the program, those selected had, in addition, a strong motivation to accept methadone treatment. In one group of applicants, only

521 heroin addicts out of 1,233 applicants were selected for treatment. The addicts accepted into the program were required to seek employment, to abstain from illicit drug use, and to refrain from criminal or antisocial behavior. Substantial numbers were discharged from the program.

A *single daily dose of methadone prevents withdrawal and drug hunger*. This claim was the basis for the enthusiasm with which methadone was distributed in maintenance clinics. In fact, it is not the drug that makes only a single daily dose necessary and prevents withdrawal symptoms and the rush, but rather the method by which the clinics dispense it. Oral administration of methadone dissolved in fruit juice allows it to be absorbed slowly into the bloodstream. Oral administration of other opiates produces the same results. Slow absorption produces only mild euphoric peaks and stretches the drug's effects over a twelve-hour period, as opposed to intravenous injection, which produces a sudden rush, followed in a few hours by depression and withdrawal symptoms.

Methadone blocks the effects of other opiates. It was once thought that methadone had the ability to block the effects of heroin. It was thought that by maintaining addicts on high enough doses of methadone, the sensual effects from taking other opiates would be blocked. Evidence has proved this is not the case.

The results of one study indicate that methadone patients use other opiates (Dobbs, 1971). The investigation was conducted using a random sample of 100 patients who were receiving methadone. Over a one-month period, urinalyses showed that 28 percent of all the addicts tested were using one of the other opiates, 70 percent of those who had been in treatment for six for eight months were using other opiates.

Many addicts in methadone treatment programs seek sensual effects not only from heroin, but from other drugs as well. One study (Taylor, 1975) tested forty patients in a methadone program for multiple drug use. After the patients had been in treatment for at least six months, 83 percent had used at least one other drug; 78 percent had used heroin; 30 percent, a barbiturate; 25 percent, an amphetamine; and 8 percent, extra methadone. At the end of fourteen months on the methadone program, 97 percent had cheated in some way. Heroin use had risen to 92 percent; barbiturate use, to 44 percent; and amphetamine use, to 69 percent.

Alcohol is one of the preferred alternative drugs to heroin for methadone patients. The wife of a methadone addict quoted in the *New York Times* (May 4, 1975) said: "Alcohol is the most widely used 'high' among methadone addicts [on maintenance doses] because when used with methadone it promotes a euphoric condition most similar to that of heroin." It has also been noted that methadone addicts become heavy users of marijuana (Fudge & Penk, 1973).

Methadone maintenance is the cheapest kind of treatment. This claim is misleading. Statistics tend to confuse legal prices with black market prices and often ignore the price of opiates on the world market. For example, it is true that in the United States the price of black market methadone is below the price of an equal dose of black market heroin. On the world market in 1971, when the methadone clinics first opened on a large scale, however, the wholesale cost of 100 milligrams of legal heroin in Southeast Asia was nine to twenty-three cents, compared with thirty cents for 100 milligrams of legal methadone in the United States. Milligram for milligram methadone costs more than heroin on the world market. If we compare equivalent doses of heroin and methadone, methadone costs even more because heroin is about two and one-fourth times stronger. If the United

States government wanted to purchase heroin on the world market, heroin would probably be cheaper to use than methadone in maintenance programs (see Appendix 3, Tables 13 and 14).

Legal maintenance programs reduce crime and eliminate the black market. It seems only logical that if addicts no longer need to hustle for money there will be a corresponding decline in drug-related crimes. But this would hold true only if methadone were used in maintenance doses and restricted to legal use. Neither of these conditions exists: there is overwhelming evidence that drugs dispensed from clinics are bought and sold illegally on the streets. The methadone dissolved in juice can be crystallized out, and methadone tablets are appearing on the street market. In fact, a black market for methadone developed within a short time of the opening of methadone clinics with the methadone diverted from legal dispensaries by clinic doctors who overprescribed and by poorly administered clinics. One former junkie said that most of the addicts entering the drug rehabilitation clinic he now attends are addicted, not to heroin, but to methadone "smuggled out of maintenance clinics by enterprising patients."

Illegally manufactured methadone is on the street market as well. Since it is a synthetic, methadone can be made in a chemistry laboratory and is often now sold on the black market as heroin. At the San Francisco Haight-Ashbury Medical Clinic, it was reported that urine tests of 122 patients who used drugs showed that 29 had taken methadone in the previous forty-eight hours. Of these, half thought they had taken heroin.

Methadone has not been effective in curtailing drug-related crime. A study was made of 416 addicts after they had been enrolled for one year in a methadone treatment program (Epstein, 1974). Among those younger than thirty-one, the number of drug offenses and forgery and prostitution charges decreased during the year of treatment, but the number of robbery charges quadrupled, assault charges increased almost 50 percent, and burglary and property theft charges increased.

Methadone is a harmless drug. Contrary to popular opinion, methadone is as addictive as any of the other opiates and is as potentially dangerous.

Brain damage has been reported from the use of methadone. An examination of fourteen people who had died from overdoses of methadone showed that the long-term users of methadone suffered changes in their brain tissues that set off new chains of chemical processes in their bodies (Roizin *et al.*, 1972). Such evidence should discourage the use of high doses of methadone until more is known about the effects of opiates on the brain.

Case studies indicate that the effects of methadone on sexual functioning are similar to those of the other opiates. Methadone, like heroin, causes a decline in sexual capacity and disturbs the menstrual cycle and decreases the chance for conception. In fact, 75 percent of the methadone patients in one study said their sexual performance was more impaired by methadone than it had been by heroin. Their blood levels of testosterone were lower than those of either the heroin users or the controls (Cicero *et al.*, 1975). It is also true that the longer the period of addiction, the more difficult the restoration of sexual functioning.

Infants born to methadone-addicted mothers have more severe and prolonged symptoms of withdrawal than infants of mothers addicted to heroin (Kandall & Gartner, 1973), and it has been shown that infants of mothers taking maintenance doses over 100 milligrams per day are especially likely to show signs of withdrawal (Glass & Evans, 1972). The addicted infants may also have to live with a modified development of portions of the brain (those that respond to opiates) that control certain aspects of the personality.

When methadone is used indiscriminately by a person who takes multiple drugs or by someone who has not built up a tolerance, an ordinary dose can lead to death. With the increase in the illegal use of methadone, death from methadone overdose is rising. In New York City it now outranks heroin as the cause of drug deaths.

For the small children of addicted parents, there is a particular danger. Methadone is usually given to the addict in a solution of orange or grape juice, and the juice is often kept in the refrigerator within easy and tempting reach, making it all too easy for a child to receive a lethal dose of methadone. Many such fatalities are on record.

About 80,000 heroin addicts are now in methadone programs. According to one government estimate, this represents a little less than 20 percent of the heroin addicts. Another 45,000 are in treatment other than methadone programs; 85,000 are in jail; and 250,000 are on the street.

The British system

Between 1926 and 1968, British law allowed a physician willing to take an addict as a patient to prescribe narcotics as his judgment dictated. Prescriptions were filled essentially free of charge. Pharmacists were required to keep records of the narcotics dispensed. A confidential index of the "reported and known" addicts was kept in the government Home Office. This index, kept in detail since the 1930s, is still maintained. Initially, only a few hundred narcotic addicts were known to the Home Office. They used morphine, cocaine, or heroin and included doctors, nurses, elderly seamen, those who had become addicted after taking opiates to relieve severe pain.

The system, designed primarily to care for middle-aged addicts (and those willing to restrict their dose of narcotics), made it possible for addicts to lead relatively normal and useful lives. Until 1960, the program seemed to work, and the number of narcotic addicts remained stable. Then the number rose dramatically. In eight years (1960–1968) the figure went from 437 (including 94 heroin addicts) to almost 3,000. The Home Office index shows that, for a period during this time, the number of heroin users was doubling every eighteen months.

There was massive overprescription; a few physicians were reported to have prescribed as much heroin as patients demanded. For the first time, an illicit market was created as addicts sold off surplus supplies, primarily to young people who, after a few weeks, would seek a physician willing to prescribe opiates for them. In 1969 the street sources were derived almost exclusively from supplies dispensed by prescription (James, 1969). It became apparent that the long-established program for addiction, which had been effective for older addicts, would not work for young addicts who craved the sensual effects of opiates and, therefore, needed to take increasingly larger doses.

As a result of the misuse of the narcotic maintenance program, the British system was changed in 1968. Clinics for the treatment of addiction were opened. Now only the doctors associated with the clinics or with special drug treatment centers who have special licenses from the Home Office are allowed to prescribe heroin or cocaine for addicts. Morphine and methadone may still be prescribed for addicts by physicians outside the clinics, but physicians generally refer addicts to the clinics. New cases must be reported to the Home Office.

In contrast to American methadone clinics, most aspects of policy and treatment at the British drug clinics are decided by the individual clinics. The clinics vary in structure and style; it is said that there are as many systems of narcotic control in England as there are consultant psychiatrists running the clinics. For example, the prescriptions may be for daily, three times weekly, or weekly doses. In some cases the addict is given his prescription; in others, the prescription is mailed to the pharmacy. Some clinics dispense the drugs at the clinic; some give injections, some give oral doses. Some require detoxification and use maintenance doses of methadone or heroin; some prescribe liberally. Some clinics refuse to prescribe heroin for outpatients. Some clinics are attached to teaching hospitals; others are independent. Some offer extensive psychiatric and social services; others do almost nothing except provide drugs. Several approaches may be used in one clinic depending upon the needs of the individual addict. The number of addicts is kept small so that the addicts are known personally, and addicts are rarely allowed to transfer from one clinic to another.

The British annual statistical data on drug addiction are recognized as the best and most detailed in the world and are frequently used in studies of drug abuse. The British figures on opiate addicts are often quoted in the United States as evidence for the success of the British clinic program in reducing heroin use. The Home Office figures show that in 1967, the year before the clinic program was started in England, 1,299 people were taking only heroin. By 1972 the number had dropped to 867. However, during the same period, those taking only methadone climbed from 243 to 2,171. Furthermore, since the opening of the clinic program, 70 percent of the outpatients taking methadone have been prescribed a form suitable for injection. Evidently many heroin users preferred or were switched by the physicians to injectable methadone. Some interpret the above statistics to mean that addicts exchange or sell their prescribed methadone for illicit heroin. If this is true, heroin use did not actually decrease as much as the figures indicate.

Although the Home Office figures show that the rate of

increase in addiction to all narcotics dropped from the high of the few years preceding the opening of the clinics, the number of new addicts is still increasing. Illicit methadone and Chinese heroin are now on the streets, and the number of convictions for drug offenses is rising (Johnson, 1975). Convictions for the use of the manufactured drugs (morphine, cocaine, heroin, and synthetic opiates including methadone) rose from 37 in 1955 to 1,359 in 1969 and to 2,068 in 1972. As in other countries, English heroin users are also using barbiturates, amphetamines, and tranquilizers.

The English are questioning the benefits of having added another legal opiate to the market. Many British physicians prescribed injectable methadone before it was clear that only oral administration prevented withdrawal symptoms with only one daily dose and that the drug did not block the effect of heroin. The patients who switched from opiate injection to oral methadone benefited. Those who switched from injection of another opiate to methadone injections probably did not. Some clinic directors have said that methadone is the worst borrowing they could have made from the United States (Judson, 1974).

Drawbacks of maintenance and substitution

It is virtually impossible to set up maintenance programs that take into account short- and long-range benefits for both the addict and society. Many questions have no simple answers. At what age should we administer an opiate? Do we maintain addicts under eighteen on opiates? Do we give oral doses for their longer lasting effects or the intravenous injections preferred by the addict? If given intravenously, do we dispense five doses a day to prevent the opiate from getting on the black market or do we trust the addict with a day's supply? What dose should be given: the higher dose in an attempt to keep the addict from buying street drugs, or the lower dose with less chance of physical and mental damage? What about the drop in price of illegal opiates when the opiate is made legal? Will not the black market still be more convenient? If heroin addicts are unwilling to restrict themselves to maintenance doses of methadone, have we gained anything by giving them another addiction?

Scientists continue to seek drugs that will block the sensual effects of opiates and will not produce the sensual or side effects. Cyclazocine, nalozone, and EN-1639A are such drugs and are now being used experimentally. They can block some effects of opiate addiction. However, they have some unpredictable and undesirable side effects; few prevent and some actually precipitate withdrawal symptoms. More research is needed before they are used in drug treatment programs.

I believe that there is little prospect of ever finding a drug to cure drug addiction. No drug can precisely duplicate natural controls, and no drug can exactly cancel effects of another. To be truly effective, the antagonist drug must reverse all the undesirable effects of the opiates on each of many sites of action without damaging the natural functions. There is probably little chance that such a drug will be found.

My main concern about maintenance programs is that the longer the addict remains on opiates, the harder it is to stop using them and return to normal. The follow-up studies of drug users in the U.S. Army showed that heroin users could give up heroin and recover if they stopped early in their use. For confirmed addicts who are unable to give up opiates, opiate maintenance programs allow them to return to a useful, but still restricted life. These programs, however, should not be offered to all addicts. Indeed, many addicts are unaware of (or have forgotten) what it was like to be completely drug-free, or they are too frightened or apprehensive to try. It seems unfair to the addict to offer him opiates to prolong his habit and harden his dependency, when, if relieved of this burden at an early stage, he will recover from his sensory deprivation. As one medical investigator who had taken heroin regularly for two weeks as an experiment said: "It's a month now since we stopped the stuff. . . . It's been wonderful to feel fit and to relish life again" (Oswald, in Judson, 1974). To maintain the young on drugs that diminish their ability to enjoy life fully seems tragic when there are alternatives.

We must be sure, therefore, that drug clinics are not merely dispensing drugs, but are giving addicts every help and encouragement to get off drugs as early in drug use as possible. We also must be sure that maintenance programs are not creating addicts.

We must not be so eager to solve the social problems of increasing drug use – such as the increase in crime – or to feel that "something is being done" about the drug problem that we overlook what is best for the addict and for society in the long run. Rehabilitation to a drug-free life is difficult for the addict, for his family, and for society as a whole. The short-term cost of rehabilitation may be greater than that of maintenance, but the cost both in dollars and in wasted human potential will be even greater if we encourage opiate use for those who could become drug-free.

CHAPTER 9

Mind expansion

Throughout the preceding chapters, we have tried to explain how sensual drugs diminish the power of the brain to function in a normal, healthy way. This is an important argument against drugs, for it is only through our brains that we can give our lives meaning.

Not many of us, though, can say that we use our mental powers to their fullest. Although evolution has expanded the physical capacity of our minds over that of our animal ancestors, thus endowing us with much greater potential for thinking, our minds are seldom trained to use even close to their full capacity. The potential for expanding our minds exists in almost all of us; we have within us the means of increasing our usefulness, satisfaction, and enjoyment of life.

Those who reduce the power of their brains reduce their capacities for pleasure and meaning in their lives. The addict suffering sensory deprivation is passive and unresponsive. Information comes into his brain from his senses, but his brain cannot integrate and interpret it properly. If he is to restore his body and mind, he must care for the needs of both. He must eat properly and get enough exercise and rest. He must practice using his mind, thereby becoming more sensitive to his surroundings, and retrain his brain to use sensory information, memory, associations, and reason to rediscover gratification, pleasure, and health.

Since the brain works on the pleasure principle, a person whose needs are satisfied is not likely to seek the artificial and transient pleasure of sensual drugs. By the same principle, how strongly an addict is motivated to redevelop his mental powers depends on how much pain he feels at the loss of his natural satisfaction and pleasure. Unfortunately, the veil of a drug-oriented life style obscures the limitations sensual drugs impose on the mind.

Although mind expansion is only one aspect of rehabilitation, it is singled out because it is an area in which the rehabilitating addict can begin to experience gratification early in the process. He can work at his own pace and in the direction he personally finds most helpful.

I have found that addicts readily comprehend mind expansion when it is explained in terms of *biofeedback*. Feedback is the process by which the brain (or any instrument initiating a command) determines how well a command is carried out and makes adjustments to bring about the desired result. All the regulative functions of the body, whether conscious or subconscious, depend on the principles of feedback. The brain is fed information through the nervous system from all the millions of receptors in the body. Information is also fed to the brain by its own mechanisms of memory and association. When the brain issues a command, these receptors return information on how the command is carried out so that the brain can make adjustments to carry out its command smoothly and efficiently.

A thermostat is a good mechanical example of feedback. When the thermostat is set at the desired temperature and the temperature falls below that setting, a device switches an electrical signal that turns on the heater. When the temperature rises above the set temperature, the feedback to the heater is interrupted by the thermostat, and the heat supply is turned off.

The principle of feedback is essential to the learning process. Naturally, the feedback system in the body is more complicated than a mechanical one; there are many separate feedback controls for each function, arranged and coordinated so that the degree of control is fine, smooth, and firm whether the activity is small or large. Through feedback the brain explores, integrates, and adjusts to a situation by using old mental patterns of thought or by forming new ones. This can be observed in the infant as he encounters and masters new situations.

In training or retraining the body's feedback systems, functions that are well below the immediate control of the consciousness are continually monitored and modified to conform to mental commands. In this way, functions that are controlled subconsciously are eventually brought into the range of conscious command. Even though the functions remain subconscious activities, they indirectly respond to the will. Interestingly, once the movement learned through this process is perfected, the command and response become subconscious. The movement becomes automatic.

This is clear in many learning activities. In learning to type, for example, there is a long struggle to establish the right associational pathways. Once they are established, the typist no longer needs to think about the placement of each finger or of separate letters; the motions fall into place as he thinks the words. The skilled diver spends long periods on the springboard adjusting the sequence of his body's movements according to the discerning eye of his trainer, who provides the needed input for the diver. With this feedback, the diver makes the necessary adjustments to perfect moves that eventually become automatic.

Feedback loops for body movements are trained from infancy. The infant learns to command compliance from the muscles of eyes first, then the hands, and, at a much later stage, the legs for walking. Each of these is as complicated as the task of diving. In old age, partly owing to decay in the nervous system, some of the feedback loops fail so that much coordination that was once smooth and steady becomes intermittently strong and weak, as secondary feedback loops attempt to take over when the established feedback pathways begin to fail. This results in tremor. In decay of the nervous system, an interruption of the feed-back process is more likely to occur than is the complete disruption of motor command that takes place with paralysis.

Much of learning, then, depends on the feedback system. Through it the diver, the typist, and the infant establish nerve pathways that are conditioned to give a certain response on command – a perfect dive, a letter free of errors, a coordinated crawl. The longer we can keep the feedback system working in top condition, the more fully we can direct our lives. It is through training and effort that our minds can be expanded.

We have been discussing biological feedback in its most fundamental sense. Recently scientists have made dis-coveries that give a new, more specific meaning to the term biofeedback.

The brain's controls below the consciousness have always used a feedback system to monitor such functions as heartbeat, blood pressure, and body temperature. Now, through biofeedback machines, scientists are discovering that these functions can also be controlled by the conscious brain. (Followers of Yoga and Zen Buddhism have long known how to control these involuntary functions con-sciously.) Biofeedback machines monitor functions and supply the brain with feedback information. The subject is hooked up to equipment that can translate his body func-tions into lights, graphs, or sounds. He concentrates on trying to control the light or sound. He is not asked to raise or lower his blood pressure or temperature directly, but rather to keep the tone low, the lights off, or the needle moving on the machine. He keeps his mind on the monitor, not on the body function itself. It has been found, in fact, that if the subject tries to affect the body function directly, his performance, recorded on the machine, is worse. The conditioning has allowed some subjects to control inner functions without using the machine as a monitor. Many have even learned to increase the amount of α-waves in their brains. These waves, associated with states of calm and meditation, are the easiest to bring under control.

Laboratory experiments have demonstrated certain medical applications of the machine for patients with high blood pressure and heart difficulties, and it has been used to treat anxiety, headache, insomnia, and loss of muscle control. Some of its future uses may be in psychotherapy, in the treatment of pain and epileptic seizure, and in treatment of paralyzed muscles and poor circulation. A study of the brain's hemispheres (Galin & Ornstein, 1975) has suggested that biofeedback may also be useful in improving thought performance. By monitoring the hemispheres with biofeedback equipment, a subject may be able to learn to strengthen the pathways between his brain's right and left hemispheres.

There is apparently a great potential for the biofeedback machines, but their use is mainly in the experimental stage. Some machines are available on the market, but they should be used only under medical supervision. We do not really know what long-term harm might result from upsetting the synchronization of the internal body rhythms by altering the internal functions. Individual responses to such tampering can vary. For example, for some people, α-waves reflect anxiety, so that increasing α-waves voluntarily would be disadvantageous and even dangerous. Psychosomatic illnesses are as likely to be aggravated as helped by altering the state of the inner functions. Until the limits of control are defined, biofeedback machines should be used with caution. The brain's control over functions of the autonomic nervous system is apparently protected – protected for some good reason.

I have mentioned biofeedback machines only to indicate possibilities for expanding the brain. Conscious being depends on what the brain does with the information that reaches it through the senses, the smooth muscles, and evaluations and thoughts initiated in the brain itself. What we become, therefore, depends on what we feed into the brain. Whether we choose to give unlimited information to the brain or whether we deprive it and thus thwart the mind's ability to function and expand is up to us. Whether we get pleasure and satisfaction from sensory information and from our thoughts and whether we make positive or negative associations to store in memory for future use is up to us. Of course, we do not control *all* the brain's activities, but as we have seen, the line between conscious and subconscious control is proving to be even more difficult to draw than was formerly thought. The mind has a tremendous ability to expand its power, though in most of us this power lies dormant.

It is not that the brain actually expands – new brain cells cannot be grown – but more is made of what is there. New pathways through the brain can be formed or weak pathways reinforced. Watching someone who is recovering from a brain injury that has affected his motor control, one can almost "see" the pathways form as the injured brain gradually manages to coordinate its functioning again. We have all experienced a breakthrough, though on a smaller scale, when solving a difficult problem. The brain can be likened to a cavern: some paths and tunnels are well worn and lead to well-known chambers; other chambers can be reached only by barely passable tunnels or by opening new routes. As new areas are explored, new adjoining areas are exposed. There is almost no limit to the potentials for mind expansion.

There are countless ways of expanding brain power without resorting to mechanical monitors. We have seen these dramatically illustrated in rehabilitated addicts; but the methods are essentially the same for addicts and nonaddicts alike.

We all can learn a lesson from the ex-addict. After he is detoxified, he must relearn how to use his mind; he must gradually force himself to explore his world, to reach out to other people, and to seek new interests. Becoming interested in food, nature, or people affords fascinations whose study could fill a lifetime. The ex-addict *must* put himself in a position to use his brain; he must expose it to new and interesting situations where it is forced to use information from all the senses. Thus he can become fully aware of sights, sounds, smells, tastes, and touch.

Researchers have recently reported that brain-injured rats recover much faster in "enriched cages" full of games, ladders, and blocks than in well-cared-for but "impoverished" cages. The rats that received a two-hour daily exposure to the enriched cages benefited as much as rats that had been in the enriched settings for twenty-four hours a day. The implication is clear: the brain can recover from injury, but it needs stimulation to do so (Rosenzweig *et al.*, 1975).

It does not cost anything or depend on travel to learn to see, not just look, and to listen, not just hear. Anyone can develop his senses through conscious effort. For example, a blind man develops acute senses of hearing, touch, and smell; the musician, a sense of hearing; the wine taster, senses of taste and smell; the gymnast, a sense of balance and muscle control. The former drug user can learn to do the same. He must learn and practice to use, not ignore, the information that comes into the brain from the senses.

Some people get less from experiences than others. A person may go into an art museum and remark upon leaving: "I saw it all and every piece was the same." Obviously, perception is, to a large extent, a matter of experience and training. Natural powers of perception are of a relatively low magnitude unless they are developed. I witnessed a superb example of people ignoring their environment when I was traveling through Glacier National Park. A bumper-to-bumper stream of cars moved slowly and continuously on the Road to the Sun and to the top of Logan Pass. Most drivers were apparently satisfied with the restricted view from their cars and were perhaps conditioned to ignore the odor of exhaust fumes from the congestion of cars. Only a few stopped to examine the view from the mountain-top knoll close by. Those few who did stop were thrilled by the magnificence of the scenery; but of those who stopped, even fewer bothered to explore the unusually beautiful meadows within easy walking distance of the Logan Pass vantage point. Perception of anything requires effort. All of us could develop our capacities for awareness, but few of us bother to try.

The sources of pleasure and the stimuli for the expansion of the mind are almost everywhere. Even the dung beetle can provide moments of lively interest to an observer. No one tires of sunsets or sunrises. The mind is naturally curious, and curiosity can be expanded by experiences and thoughts. Experiences are expanded by repetition and by understanding of the event.

One of the greatest problems a drug addict has is in his relationships with other people. He is paranoid and thinks that others, often those closest to him, do not care, do not like him, or persecute him. He isolates himself from others and even from himself. His rehabilitation requires learning to relate to other people again, and this involves developing new pathways in the brain or rediscovering the use of old ones. The addict must learn to become genuinely interested in other people's activities, problems, and pleasures. He must expand his mind.

Once again, we can all learn to do what the addict must learn to do. When we see a friendly smile, we are, in fact, receiving positive feedback, and we feel pleasure. If there are few friendly faces, we need to make the overtures, and others eventually respond. This cements friendships and brings understanding, sympathy, and love. It can be gratifying to see how far this kind of effort can reach.

In addition to external sources of stimulation that expand the mind, the brain can be its own source. We can receive pleasure from memories, associations, and thoughts. Solving difficult problems is often rewarding and is certainly an expanding experience. The ability to change mood through thought alone is particularly important to the addict who has relied on drug-induced moods. Positive thinking can lead to understanding, forgiveness, the ability to give and accept love and affection, a sense of belonging, lack of embarrassment, patience, enthusiasm, and willingness to be responsible for one's self.

Religion is a powerful force for directing thought, exploring one's inner self, and establishing spiritual values. Religion has special importance for the rehabilitating addict, since, as discussed in Chapter 8, the capacity for religious response remains in spite of drug-induced sensory deprivation.

Abrahamsen, a psychiatrist and author of many books on the use of the mind, includes ethical and spiritual values as necessary components of emotional maturity. His book, *The Road to Emotional Maturity*, although written in 1958, is still a good, basic source on the subject, and is presented in simple, clear language. In it he includes an especially useful list of stumbling blocks to emotional maturity. He says that the sources within ourselves are the only reliable sources of security; that we can use these inner forces to draw out our constructive abilities and help bring tranquility to our minds. "Remember," he says, "that you have powerful forces within yourself which can help you."

Mind expansion gives us greater control over our lives and enables us to live more fully and happily. This is especially important for the drug addict, who has lost much of his ability to sense what is around him.

The pleasures of sensual drugs may be immediate, but they are not gratifying or sustained, and they are not greater than those induced naturally. Drugs do not give a real high or expand the mind. As one ex-user expressed it, drugs stimulate, but they reduce the ability to feel. The mind is not expanded, but limited; the addict essentially ends his mental growth. Natural stimulation, on the other hand, can expand the mind to give pleasure and gratification that does not fade with use, but is reinforced by it.

It is especially important for a rehabilitating addict to experience what one psychologist calls "achievement" feedback (McClelland, 1965). Goals should be set high enough so the mind is expanded, but some should be within easy reach so there can be a continuous sense of satisfaction.

No single formula can be given for the expansion of the mind. What may be meaningful to one person may not be to another. One may have a wide range of interests; another, more intense interests in a few areas; some may prefer physical activity to mental activity. Whatever direction one chooses, it must be remembered that the growth of the mind takes effort and time. Everything is opened up by growth: the taste of food, the sounds of music, the smells of nature, the feel of wood, clay, or soft wool can all be explored. Through the senses, one can become aware of the warmth of the sun; the stimulation from a deep breath of fresh air; the satisfaction of a yawn or a stretch; the pleasure from the smile of another. One can develop the capacity for sensual enjoyment through learning, reading, talking, and working. There is no end of possibilities for expanding the mind. One can get satisfaction from athletics, from a hard task well performed, or from control of inner functions. Feedback is everywhere, but one must be sensitive to it. A person can have a zest for life, be interested in people and things, and continue to grow throughout his life if he uses the power available in his own brain. The search for ethical and spiritual values, study, thought, and communication are the clearest paths to realizing the full potential of the brain.

CHAPTER 10

Marijuana

Marijuana is the most controversial of the sensual drugs. Because short-term use seemed to have little adverse effect and because, until quite recently, little was known about how the drug affected body chemistry, it was assumed that marijuana was like other well-tolerated drugs and medications. It seemed less harmful than other sensual drugs, and incidents of lethal overdose were rare. The fact that it was referred to as a "mild" hallucinogen reinforced the idea that it was harmless.

The truth is that in the 1960s, when marijuana first became popular, the public was unaware of the consequences of its use. The fad was new, and users had not yet experienced the long-term effects. "Authorities" appeared on every side, each contradicting the others. Alarmists exaggerated the negative evidence; optimists preached the safety and benefits of marijuana use. The fact that users could not see the harm marijuana smoking was doing them complicated the issue. The facts, however, now rest on a firm scientific base; we now know some of the chemistry of the cannabis drugs and something of how they affect the body organs and cell functions.

Marijuana is not a new drug. Cannabis (the botanical name for the hemp plant) has been used since the tenth

214

century A.D. The drug is in the resinous wax of the hemp plant and is produced by secretory glands resembling hollow hairs that extend from the surface of the leaves. At the tip of each hair is a microscopic droplet of solidified resin. Crudely separated resin is called hashish. In the few countries where it is legal, shops supply the compressed resin in various shapes and sizes: pencil-shaped cylinders, bricks, spheres, hexagonal cakes, disks, and granules. Its color varies from amber to ebony, and it may be as hard as wax or as soft as putty. Marijuana, the dried, crumbled leaves and flowers of the hemp plant, is rated according to appearance, potency, and origin. The hemp plant's resin is a pesticide; it is harmful to the nervous systems of insects and animals.

In the United States in the 1930s, marijuana came to public attention because of its endemic use in Harlem and New Orleans. Around 1950 it became part of a movement among artists and intellectuals, the followers of Aldous Huxley, who rediscovered old literature and wrote works of their own describing the pleasures of cannabis drugs. In the 1960s Timothy Leary began to write and lecture on the benefits of the "mind-expanding" drugs (including psilocybin and LSD). It was to both these old and modern literary sources that people went to confirm that marijuana use was safe and beneficial. Accounts of the long-term, harmful effects of cannabis drugs reported by the Indian Hemp Drugs Commission in 1894 and by Chopra and Chopra in 1939 were ignored or discounted.

The epidemic use of marijuana in the 1960s among middle-class youth aroused greater public and scientific interest in the drug. In 1965 the principal psychoactive ingredient of cannabis, Δ-9-tetrahydrocannabinol (Δ-9-THC), was isolated and identified. The purified active substance has proved indispensable in learning about the effects of marijuana. Previously we only had crude smoke or extracts from the leaves of the plant to use in experiments, and exact measurements were almost impossible to make. There are about fifty potentially active substances in marijuana. In the major group are the cannabinoids; in the subgroup are the cannabinols. The principal cannabinoid in most cannabis drugs is Δ-9-THC (infrequently classified as Δ-1-THC). However, other active substances may make minor contributions to the effects of marijuana.

In addition to the cannabinoids, cannabis drugs contain atropinelike substances (alkaloids) that may influence such body functions as blood pressure and pupil diameter. These alkaloids have definite drug properties when administered separately. It is believed, however, that the alkaloids make negligible contributions to the effects of marijuana in humans.

It is possible that the effects of marijuana differ depending on whether the drug is smoked or eaten. When it is smoked, some of the cannabinols (the acids) are converted from the inactive acid form to active THC by the high temperature. This conversion does not take place when marijuana is eaten. When marijuana is smoked, however, at least half the THC is consumed in the combustion or escapes as smoke (Agurell *et al.*, 1972).

Some of the THC absorbed into the body, whether eaten or smoked, is gradually converted into the metabolite, 11-hydroxy-THC, a substance with even greater psychoactive properties than THC. The distribution of the two substances in the body and brain, however, is similar (see Appendix 2).

Advocates of marijuana use generally say that the drug has not been proved harmful. Their arguments can be quite convincing. Many reports on the subject have been published; unfortunately, they are often conflicting and confusing. Studies have been reviewed by individuals or groups who would be expected to give objective evaluations. Inaccuracies occur, however, either through lack of understanding or intentional bias. The fact is no scientific evidence has been found to prove that marijuana is safe; we have only the personal testimonies of short-term users.

Very small concentrations of THC can affect cells. A few exposures are certainly nothing to worry about; but because THC is retained and accumulated in the body, prolonged, regular use may damage body cells. Brain changes, lung damage, decline in male hormone production, chromosome alterations, and depressed cell division all can occur.

The list of altered functions that can be observed in marijuana users is long: changes in personality, memory, facial expression, thought formation, mood, motivation, skin color, and motor coordination. The user, however, can seldom see these changes in himself.

The evidence against marijuana is coming in from all over the world, and we are now in a position to answer questions concerning its effects. In the pages that follow, I will answer some of the questions most often asked about marijuana use.

Does marijuana alter brain function?

Marijuana affects the perception of time, distance, and speed. It upsets motor coordination, causing unsteady hands, a change in gait, uncontrolled laughter, and a lag between thought and facial expressions. Sexual functions can be disturbed. Short-term memory deteriorates. In the early stages of use, some users suffer from nausea, vomiting, and diarrhea. Users may find that when they are high the whites of their eyes and facial skin become red; that their pupils dilate and become sensitive to light; that their appetites increase or decrease markedly; that their mouths and throats seem dry; and that their extremities grow cold. What all these effects have in common is that they result from changes in the brain's control centers, located deep in the brain.

Deep brain functions, though subconscious, cannot be

separated from conscious thought processes. The deep relay centers feed information to the controlling mechanisms of the consciousness. Thus, when marijuana disturbs functions centered in the deep control centers, disorienting changes in the mind occur. The user's psychomotor coordination is impaired. He may suffer illusions and hallucinations, difficulty in recalling events in the immediate past, slowed thinking and narrowed attention span, depersonalization, euphoria or depression, drowsiness or insomnia, difficulty in making accurate self-evaluation, a lowering of inhibition, a loss of judgment, and mental and physical lethargy.

The relationship between brain functions and the use of marijuana is being more and more fully documented. Heath (1972*a*, 1973) found that brain wave patterns in the septal region (in the limbic system) were altered after subjects had taken marijuana. Recordings were made of brain waves from sites deep in the brains of both humans and monkeys where the principal mental effects of the drug are produced. Subjects were then exposed to hemp drugs while deep electrodes recorded electrical potentials in various parts of the limbic region:

The monkeys developed immediate changes in behavior and brain wave activity from some deep brain sites. With the passage of time, these monkeys . . . developed persisting changes in brain activity. These changes outlasted the immediate period of an hour or two after the conclusion of the smoking and were found to be present up to five days later. Those monkeys exposed to inactive marijuana, that is with the active ingredient, THC, removed, showed neither acute nor chronic effects. [Heath, in U.S. Senate Hearings, 1974]

Critics objected that the doses given to the monkeys in this experiment were too high to be applied instructively. The objection can be overcome by adjusting the doses according to a standard formula for relating the doses given to animals of different sizes. Once the adjustment is made, Heath estimates the moderate doses received by his monkeys were equivalent to one marijuana cigarette per day for humans, based on a cigarette of 1.5 grams of 3 percent Δ-9-THC; the heavy doses, below the average daily dose used by the heavy hashish smokers in the U.S. Army in Germany; and the light doses, equivalent to one-half a marijuana cigarette per day for humans (see Appendix 9 and under "Relation of animal and human studies," below).

Heath's studies of brain waves of human subjects show that marijuana has selective effects on human pleasure centers as well. The immediate effects of smoking marijuana are pleasurable emotional responses and the simultaneous generation of brain waves centered in the pleasure area of the brain. These brain waves are similar to those evoked by normal activities that stimulate the pleasure centers. In one subject, the recordings made during marijuana intoxication were significantly different from those obtained during tobacco, alcohol, or amphetamine use. The changes in recordings with marijuana were distinct, whereas the changes in recordings with the other drugs were minimal or absent. This suggests that sensual drugs have varying degrees of effect and may influence different pleasure centers.

Heath has described the areas of the limbic region affected by marijuana smoke as relay centers for sensory perception and emotional response. When the functions of these centers are impaired, the user experiences hallucinations and other forms of altered perceptions common to schizophrenia and drug-induced intoxications. Another study traced radioisotope-labeled THC in the brains of monkeys to observe its distribution. The drug was highly concentrated in the frontal lobes and the hippocampal area of the limbic region. The authors of this study found it "tempting to suggest that the interaction between these two areas plays an important part in associating stimuli into a temporal context. It is well known that one of the chief effects of marijuana is distortion of time perception" (McIsaac *et al.*, 1971).

These observations of selective uptake led to further research. Animal experiments have established that THC uptake is greater in the gray matter (the cerebral cortex and deep brain area) than in the white matter. Clinical findings have linked suppression of frontal lobe function with marijuana use (Powelson, in U.S. Senate Hearings, 1974; personal communication). The frontal lobe area is the center for abstract thinking. Powelson found that marijuana can cause "marijuana thinking," in which abstract reasoning is dissociated from the concrete. Encephalography, performed to explore the effects of heavy and prolonged use of cannabis, disclosed cerebral atrophy in the deep brain area in ten consecutively seen young men severely affected by cannabis (Campbell *et al.*, 1971).

It has been established that THC accumulates in and alters the fatty structures of cell membranes (Paton *et al.*, 1972; Paton, 1975). These fatty materials are vital parts of the membrane's functional structure. THC accumulates at the fat interface and causes the film of fatty material to be restructured. This also affects the fine, specialized structures of the cell surface through which one brain cell communicates with another.

Much research has been done on the manifestations of altered brain function in the user. In his testimony before the U.S. Senate hearings on the marijuana and hashish epidemic (1974), Malcolm discussed three features of marijuana use: suggestibility, the amotivational syndrome, and ideological conflict. He noted that when emotional responses and sensory information are distorted, critical judgment is impaired and users may become more vulnerable to external evaluations and suggestions. He observed a loss of will and conscious control. These effects can be pronounced during the marijuana high. They also persist after the period of acute intoxication and accumulate with chronic use; there is a logical relation between these effects and the amotivational state of the habitual user.

The "motivational" effect of marijuana as reported from recent studies done in Jamaica, Greece, and Costa Rica should, perhaps, be explained here. Some chronic marijuana users report that they feel a burst of energy after taking the drug. This effect can occur only when the user's brain mechanisms have become adjusted to function in the presence of the drug; therefore, the motivational effect should not be considered as evidence contradicting the observations of researchers in these countries who have studied the long-term amotivational effect of marijuana use.

In a study in Maryland (Miliman *et al.*, 1976), hundreds of drug addicts from high schools, universities, prisons, and drug programs were studied for six to nine years. The researchers observed thought disorders in the chronic marijuana users that they identified as the *cannabis syndrome*. A major thought disorder of this syndrome was found to be "diminished drive, lessened ambition, decreased motivation, and apathy." I have observed that users often cannot recognize the amotivational effect in themselves except in retrospect. They usually notice that they have recovered their sense of motivation six to eight weeks after they give up marijuana.

Chronic suppression of mental function was also noted in a study of young Egyptians who were long-term users (Soueif, 1971). In this study, 650 cannabis users were matched to a control group. The users did poorly in comparison with the control group in all tests of mental function, even though they were not intoxicated at the time of evaluations. When the groups were compared by educational level, the greatest disparity in test performance was between the best-educated users and nonusers. Even among the illiterates studied, cannabis users had less adequate short-term memories than their matched control group.

It has also been found that mental tasks requiring attention to both procedures and goals are affected by marijuana (Clark *et al.*, 1970; Melges *et al.*, 1974). Melges reported that a cigarette containing 20 milligrams of THC (equivalent to one 2 percent cigarette – a common dose), smoked in ten minutes brought on paranoid delusions in four of his six subjects, none of whom had a history of such delusions. In other controlled studies, doses of THC comparable to low doses (5 milligrams) taken by smokers were found to affect some measured mental and motor performances (Manno *et al.*, 1970; Kiplinger *et al.*, 1971).

The effects of marijuana vary, of course, with the well-being, maturity, previous experience, and mental health of the individual; with the strength of the marijuana; and with what the user expects from the experience. Response can vary radically: at one extreme are the users who have a natural resistance; at the other are those in whom marijuana can produce a state of acute psychosis or panic. It has been claimed that such reactions occur only in those who are latent psychotics. However, Zeidenberg, a psychiatrist at Columbia University, has concluded from his studies of marijuana users that "there is no doubt that a single dose of THC can cause an acute psychotic reaction in mentally healthy individuals. One of our subjects (given THC orally) had an acute paranoid break lasting several hours. This young man is of unquestionably sound mental health" (Zeidenberg, in U.S. Senate Hearings, 1974). In conducting my research, I interviewed an athlete who became deranged from a short-term exposure to marijuana. He recovered when he stopped taking the drug. This, of course, is an example of the most severe disturbance induced by marijuana. It is apparent, however, that both the mild and severe personality and behavioral changes are the result of altered brain function.

Are marijuana-induced brain changes reversible?

Destroyed brain cells cannot be replaced. Nevertheless, the brain can readjust and recover from cell damage, chemical imbalance, or psychic upset. Damaged cells can be repaired; alternate pathways around destroyed cells can be formed through the brain; and up to a point, adjustments can be made to compensate for chemical disturbances.

How much overt cell damage or chemical upset occurs in the brain of any individual is difficult to assess, since it is both hazardous and impractical to examine the living brain. Whether the brain has recovered from the disturbance can be judged only from the visible effects.

In the early stages of marijuana use, brain disturbances appear to be completely reversible. Recovery cannot take place, however, in a few days or even a few weeks because the accumulated cannabinoids are eliminated from the tissue so slowly (see Appendix 2). Recovery may also be slowed by the fact that the brain's mechanisms, having become accustomed to stimulation by marijuana, take time to work well again.

Heavy use over a long period can cause permanent changes in the brain. It has been found, for instance, that the brains of young heavy users of cannabis can atrophy (Campbell *et al.*, 1971). The loss of brain substance was comparable to that normally found in people seventy to ninety years old. Progressive brain atrophy could certainly explain the psychic changes that occur after heavy, long-term use. The ten subjects in the study were young men who had taken cannabis daily for from three to eleven years. They had no preexisting conditions that might have produced cerebral atrophy at an early age. Shrinkage of cerebral structures was measured by roentgenographic examination of the brain after the fluid of the inner cavity of the brain had been withdrawn and replaced with air.

The study has been criticized because of the limited number of cases involved and because the subjects had used other drugs. The results, however, showed that all ten subjects had cerebral atrophy, and the fact remains that cannabis was the only drug used by all ten subjects. The correlation between the level of cannabis use and the degree of brain atrophy was high. Furthermore, the other drugs used, with the exception of alcohol, are not known to cause cerebral atrophy, whereas animal studies have shown that cannabis can cause atrophy. Alcohol could have contributed to the atrophy in two cases (Evans, 1974), but not even heavy drinking has been shown to cause cerebral atrophy in such young persons.

In a review of the work, one of the researchers of the Campbell studies (Evans, 1974) said: "Our findings were positive and disturbing. . . . The findings are consistent with cerebral destruction near the ventricles where a minor degree of atrophy is liable to produce profound effects on personality and mental functions." He concluded: "It seems to us therefore that our results call for urgent investigation of the possibility that regular heavy smoking of cannabis resin may produce cerebral atrophy."

The fact that such a difficult and dangerous study has not been repeated is no reason to discount the findings. Even one case of cannabis-linked atrophy would be cause for concern; but when examination of ten consecutive patients shows the same unusual results (according to the norm of clinical findings, unexplained brain atrophy occurs only once in 500 young persons), the evidence should be taken seriously. Statistically it is highly significant.

The best confirmation of the Campbell findings comes from Heath (in U.S. Senate Hearings, 1974). Heath studied brain waves in monkeys and humans. Monkeys with electrodes implanted deep in their brains were regularly given specific doses of active marijuana. About three months after the experiment had begun, the monkeys began to show altered brain function. Heath stated: "It appears that [the effects] are persistent, but to say they were permanent requires the passage of time and further investigation." At autopsy about a year later, the brains of the monkeys given high and intermediate doses showed significant organic damage. The ventricles had enlarged, indicating brain atrophy, and distinct changes were observed in the synapses (see Appendix 9).

Other researchers have found evidence of major organic brain changes in rats exposed to doses of THC equivalent to normal daily human doses (Rosenkrantz *et al.*, 1975; Luthra *et al.*, 1975). They noted dramatic changes in water balance and brain enzymes and a decrease in the RNA in the cerebral hemispheres (Appendix 9).

The slow recovery and the point of permanent impairment from toxic brain changes have been described in the clinical studies of Kolansky & Moore (1972*b*). They concluded from their study of individuals who were sensitive to marijuana and who used it regularly and heavily, that major changes in behavior and attitudes reflect permanent brain damage.

Miras (1967), who studied brain waves of marijuana users who smoked at least two cigarettes of marijuana a day for two years or more, found that abnormal brain wave readings corresponded to behavioral changes. In some long-term users, chronic lethargy and loss of inhibition were observed two years after the last use of marijuana. This was felt to be an indication of significant and lasting organic brain change.

These studies indicate that persistent, if not permanent, brain changes are associated with high doses and prolonged exposure to marijuana. What has not been established is the limit of exposure that permits recovery. The nature of other brain injuries, however, suggests that the extent of the damage is matched to behavioral changes and is already severe when it is detected in altered brain waves.

Does marijuana affect other body functions?

The brain is the master control for all the functions of the body. A disturbance in any of the brain's controls can affect other control systems in the body. Tremor, reddening of the eyes and dilation of the pupils, increased urine formation, increased pulse and blood pressure, and changes in blood flow pattern are all effects of changes in the brain. Besides the indirect effects of altered brain controls, it now appears that marijuana can also have a direct effect on various systems in the body. Because body functions and brain controls are interrelated, however, it cannot be precisely determined which effects of marijuana are caused by the action of the drug on the brain and which are caused by the action of the drug directly on other parts of the body.

As we have discussed, THC has an affinity for fatty structures – especially the cell membranes. Thus cells exposed to the highest blood flow are particularly vulnerable to the toxic effects of marijuana. I was the first person to measure the patterns of regional blood flow in the body (Jones, 1950, 1951). My research showed that the brain does not have uniform blood flow. I found that the most vascular part (18 percent) of the brain receives a blood flow (1.4 volumes of blood per volume of tissue per minute) four times that of the remaining 82 percent of the brain. We now know that the areas of highest blood flow in the brain are the cerebral cortex and the deep brain area and that these are the two areas in the brain most affected by marijuana exposure. I measured the blood flow in the brain, endocrine glands, liver, spleen, intestines, kidneys, heart, and bone marrow; although they constitute 10 percent of body weight, I found they receive 80 percent of the blood pumped from the left side of the heart when a person is at rest. The lungs have the highest blood flow of any tissues of the body because the entire output of blood pumped from the right side of the heart flows through the lungs. (At rest this is about 25 volumes of blood per volume of tissue per minute.) It is in these areas of high blood flow that cells are especially vulnerable because of the uptake of THC from the blood by the fat structure of cell membranes. In addition to the brain, marijuana has been observed to affect the liver and the respiratory, reproductive, and blood cell systems.

Effect on liver

The livers of animals exposed to cannabis are damaged. In humans, however, it is not clear how much of the liver damage is actually caused by marijuana and how much is caused by alcohol. In one study of marijuana users with liver damage who had also used alcohol extensively, liver function improved after abstention from alcohol. Another study found definite liver damage in human subjects who had smoked marijuana heavily for from two to eight years (Kew *et al.*, 1969). Damage was detected by a liver function test and examination of a biopsy specimen of liver tissue, using biological and electron microscope techniques. However, using the liver function test only, another researcher detected no abnormal functioning in the livers of soldiers who had used marijuana/hashish for six to fifteen months (Tennant, in U.S. Senate Hearings, 1974). It appears that liver damage takes several years rather than several months to develop and that such direct effects are cumulative and the result of long, heavy exposure. However, sensitive tests such as those used by Kew, may show that liver damage is detectable in less than several years of heavy exposure to marijuana. The high flow of blood in the liver (1 volume of blood per volume of tissue per minute) indicates the liver is vulnerable to the toxic effects of marijuana.

Effect on respiratory system

United States soldiers who smoked large amounts of marijuana/hashish for long periods showed a marked tendency toward chronic bronchitis and emphysema. In a subgroup study of thirty hashish smokers among American soldiers in Germany who consumed 25 to 30 grams of hashish per month, all were found to have chronic bronchitis. Examination of biopsy specimens established that twenty-four of the thirty had abnormal bronchial tissue. Tobacco smokers must smoke for ten to twenty years before these lung diseases develop; the symptoms appear in persons who have used hashish for only six to fifteen months (Tennant, in U.S. Senate Hearings, 1974).

The lungs of the marijuana user are more blackened by smoke than those of the tobacco smoker because, to get an effect, marijuana smoke must be inhaled deeper and held longer in the lungs. Indeed, the concentration of THC in the lungs is very much greater than in the body as a whole. Autopsy examination of the lungs of heavy marijuana smokers shows extreme breakdown in the lung structure.

It is interesting to note the reasons why marijuana must be held in the lungs. In quiet, normal breathing, fresh air is not drawn into the small air sacs, but into the smaller airway tubes (bronchioles) that ventilate the air sacs. At rest, only shallow breathing is necessary because the molecules of oxygen and carbon dioxide diffuse very rapidly between the air tubes and the air sacs. Nicotine is largely condensed on smoke particles, but these carbon particles need not be drawn into the air sacs to bring nicotine into the body. Nicotine dissociates readily from the carbon particles and enters the air sacs and blood about as readily as does oxygen. THC is different; it is tightly bound to the surfaces of carbon particles. In marijuana smoking, the smoke must be drawn, by deep inhalation, into the air sacs; breath holding allows the carbon particles to be deposited on the wall of the sacs immediately adjacent to the capillaries. Then, over a period of minutes, THC is absorbed from the carbon particles into the blood.

Table 8. *Throat and respiratory disorders associated with cannabis use*

Symptom	All cannabis users with symptom (%)	Mild cannabis users with symptom (%)	Potent cannabis users with symptom (%)
Sore throat, pharyngitis, laryngitis	39.0		
Respiratory diseases	39.0		
Chronic bronchitis	22.0	6.0	48.0
Emphysema	4.5	2.3	8.2

Source: Data from Chopra and Chopra (1939).

Hashish smokers have even more respiratory illnesses and precancerous degenerative changes of lung tissue than do marijuana smokers (Tennant, in U.S. Senate Hearings, 1974). Since hashish smokers volatilize more of the active resin with less smoke, it seems likely that the resin contains substances that are quite toxic to the respiratory passages.

Chopra and Chopra (1939) reported similar differences between the effects of mild (bhang) and potent (ganja and charas) cannabis in 1,238 users (Table 8). In 1939 when this study was done, it was not certain whether the toxic effects were due to cannabis or smoke, but more recent work on lung tissue cultures (Leuchtenberger *et al.*, 1976) has clearly established that marijuana smoke causes a greater range and degree of damage to lung cells than tobacco smoke.

Effect on endocrine system

As discussed in Chapter 2, the hypothalamus is the master endocrine gland and nerve control center; its many functions include regulating the secretion of the pituitary, which, in turn, regulates the secretions of other endocrine glands. Which effects of marijuana on endocrine functions are brought about through the hypothalamus and pituitary and which are the results of more direct effects on other endocrine controls have not yet been determined. Marijuana may actually mimic the action of certain hormones. In rats the function of the hypothalamus has been found to be disturbed by marijuana. A dose of THC administered locally in the hypothalamus of rats inhibited the pituitary-thyroid function (production of the thyroid-stimulating hormone and the thyroid hormone) (Lomax, 1970).

Kolodny *et al.* (1974) showed that testosterone, the most potent of the male sex hormones, was depressed in the blood of a group of marijuana users. Those who smoked ten or more marijuana cigarettes per week had a lower testosterone level – about two times lower than those smoking half as much marijuana. Although this study did not include people who smoked less than five marijuana cigarettes per week (or who took the drug less than four times a week or for less than six months), the significant effects, which were proportional to the degree of marijuana use, suggest that the suppression of male hormone production is about 4 percent for each marijuana cigarette smoked per week. It was also observed that sperm production in six out of the twenty subjects was significantly depressed. In those six men, there was a significant correlation between sperm count and the blood level of the pituitary hormone known to activate sperm production. The group smoking ten or more marijuana cigarettes per week had significantly less sperm and less of the pituitary hormone that controls sperm production than those smoking about half as much marijuana.

Hormone stimulation tests done on four of the marijuana smokers (using a human gonadotropic hormone extracted from placentas) showed that the testes were able to synthesize testosterone. This implies that the effect of the marijuana was centered in the brain and diminished pituitary production of both gonad-stimulating hormones (one stimulating sperm and the other sex hormone production). In three subjects who discontinued use of marijuana for two weeks, there was a pronounced, significant rise in male hormone production by the end of the first week, which continued, though less pronounced, through the second week.

In a later study, Kolodny (1975) found that there was a decline in male hormone production with short-term exposure to marijuana, but that the major decline came after more than four weeks of steady use. Other investigators have confirmed that there is a reduction in sperm count associated with marijuana use. Hembree *et al.* (1976) found a 66 percent reduction in sperm after one month of marijuana use.

In May 1974, I reported my observations on the decline in male sexuality and virility associated with marijuana smoking (in U.S. Senate Hearings, 1974). This was not a universal effect, but it occurred in a large number of users, especially those who were physically inactive. I cautioned that the effect might not be observed in vigorous, athletic young men. Subsequently, in a study of twenty-seven subjects selected for their good physical condition and good health from more than 300 marijuana-using applicants, no reduction in male hormone levels was observed (Mendelson *et al.*, 1974*b*). Although other factors may be involved, in my opinion the conclusion to be drawn from the results of both Kolodny and Mendelson is that a depression in male hormone levels occurs in *most* marijuana users, but does not necessarily occur with short-term exposure in those in the best physical condition.

Kolodny has stated that because of the effect of THC on male hormone levels, there is the possibility of other related harmful effects yet to be investigated (in U.S. Senate Hearings, 1974). At least some of the active constituents of marijuana cross the placenta and enter fetal circulation (and can also pass into breast milk). Thus, there may be a significant risk of depressed testosterone levels in the developing fetus when marijuana is used by a pregnant woman. Since normal sexual differentiation in the male embryo depends on adequate testosterone stimulation during critical stages of fetal development, maternal use of the drug may disturb that development. In rats, it has been shown that adult male behavior also depends upon the production of male hormones in utero (Gorski, 1974).

Studies of the effects of marijuana on the function of the gonads have so far been conducted only on men. However, because the gonad-stimulating hormones are controlled through the pituitary, similar changes may also be detected in women who smoke marijuana.

Some of the effects of marijuana are similar to the effects of female sex hormones. When estrogen, a female sex hormone, is administered to men, testosterone levels are depressed, breast tissue develops, secondary sex glands are affected, and sperm count decreases. These effects have been observed in male marijuana smokers. A recent experiment of spayed female rats exposed to THC (in doses that fell within the range of heavy, chronic doses used by humans) demonstrated that the effects of THC are much like the effects of estrogen. This effect was determined by the uterine weight gain in the spayed rats (Solomon *et al.*, 1976). Some of the effects of marijuana on the brain's pleasure centers may possibly be due to this estrogenlike effect. Diethylstilbestrol (DES), an artificial female hormone, has been shown to be harmful to female offspring. Given to pregnant women, this hormone increases measurably the risk that the genital tracts of female fetuses will be malformed and that female children will develop cancer of the genital tract (Herbst *et al.*, 1972).

A possible confirmation of abnormal female sex hormone influences in the cells of male hashish users has been made by Stefanis and Issidorides (1976). The white blood cells of women have a small characteristic drumstick protrusion from the cell nucleus; this structure is rarely found in white blood cells of men. This female characteristic was found by these researchers in 10 percent of the white cells from 21 out of 34 men who regularly smoked hashish. None of the nuclei in the white blood cells from the men in the control group showed drumsticks.

The effects of THC on hormone levels help explain the findings of Chopra and Chopra's study of 1,238 cannabis drug users in 1939. After an eight-year study based on interviews, the Chopras reported that 40 percent of their subjects experienced sexual depression; 16 percent reported sexual stimulation; 20 percent experienced initial stimulation and later depression; and 24 percent reported no effect. These were purely subjective reactions, but present knowledge about the variable effects of THC on hormone levels indicates that the reactions had a physiological basis. The same study investigated fertility in the 686 married or previously married subjects. Sterility was found in 2 percent of the subjects, almost double the rate in the general population.

Effect on cell function

The recent work with perhaps the broadest implications is that which shows the effect of marijuana on chromosomes, DNA, and RNA. Chromosomes carry hereditary information for each cell. The cell's genetic code passes hereditary information on both to offspring (through the egg and the sperm) and to each newly formed cell in an individual so that it (with rare exceptions) is identical to the cell from which it derives. Normal human cells, except the reproductive cells, contain forty-six chromosomes (twenty-three pairs). Hereditary information of the genetic code is carried chemically in the chromosomes by genes. The average chromosome is estimated to contain 1,000 or more genes, each carrying the genetic code in a complex molecular structure known as the DNA (deoxyribonucleic acid) molecule. DNA synthesizes another nucleic acid, ribonucleic acid (RNA), which controls all cell functions through the control of protein synthesis. Thus DNA indirectly and RNA directly control protein synthesis and therefore control cell functions.

Chromosomes are visible under the microscope. Broken chromosomes have been associated with mutations, tumors, virus disease, anemia, and the aging process. Chromosomes do break spontaneously, but at a very low rate; they break at a faster rate when exposed to radiation, certain viruses, and a few toxic chemicals, including THC.

A number of studies have established that long-term users of psychotropic drugs have a higher number of broken chromosomes than the average. There is no evidence for chromosome breakage in studies of short-term users. Initial observations suggested that chromosome damage was caused by LSD (Cohen *et al.*, 1976). Stenchever *et al.* (1974) observed that chromosome damage, including breakage, in users of psychotropic drugs is due to the use of marijuana and not to other drugs. Their study was conducted on twenty women and twenty-nine men, aged seventeen to thirty-three. Of these, twenty-seven had used only marijuana and twenty-two had used other drugs as well. Those using marijuana twice a week or more and those using it once a week or less both had significant increases in chromosome breakage. It was found that damage to chromosomes is largely independent of the intensity of the exposure, but does depend on the duration of exposure. The use of marijuana for six months to nine years (average use about three years) produced about the same degree of chromosome breakage in both light and heavy users compared with nonusers. Subjects who smoked one marijuana cigarette per day or less showed almost as much chromosome damage as those who used two or more per day. In a study of fewer subjects, chromosome breakage was found in heavy users, but not in light users (Gilmour *et al.*, 1971).

The results of another study substantiate the finding that short-term use does not result in a detectable level of chromosome breakage (Nichols *et al.*, 1974). In this study, marijuana was given in large doses to a group of users for either five or twelve days. The level of chromosome breakage in these marijuana users two and a half hours after smoking was compared with their levels just before smoking and also with their levels just prior to the five- to twelve-day test. Since Nichols did not compare regular users of marijuana with nonusers, the amount of chromosome damage from use cannot be determined from this study. The findings do indicate, however, that there is not a measurable increase in chromosome breakage in two and a half hours or over a five- to twelve-day exposure.

Chromosome breakage occurs naturally as we age and may account for some of the deterioration of aging. Even in old people, however, only a small fraction of cells have broken chromosomes. Marijuana use causes, it appears, as much chromosome damage in a few years as occurs normally in fifty years. I personally believe, however, that the debilitation commonly seen in heavy users of marijuana is due more directly to the accumulated toxic effects of THC throughout the body than to chromosome breakage. In either event, debilitation of the body does occur.

Broken chromosomes also raise a serious genetic problem. Broken chromosomes themselves are seldom a genetic hazard to offspring; damage that great cannot usually be passed on. The primary concern is that the conditions that produce broken chromosomes are also likely to damage the genes even in unbroken chromosomes. Broken chromosomes are an indication that there may also be damaged chromosomes containing mutated genes, which can be passed on to offspring. The degree of the damage is difficult to measure because the genes work in pairs, one on each paired chromosome. If one gene is malformed, the other of the pair does the work, but not completely. Nature thus provides a safety valve to protect against genetic disease; it is extremely unlikely that both genes of a pair will have been damaged. When one of a pair of genes is defective, there is usually no specific genetic disease, but rather a general decline in vigor in the offspring. Evidence of a specific gene defect has been noticed in women exposed to radiation; they produce fewer than expected male children.

After World War II, atom bomb survivors in Japan were found to have broken chromosomes in proportion to their exposure to ionizing radiation. The number of male offspring declined, which confirmed the genetic effects of damaged genes (other undetectable genetic changes undoubtedly occurred as well). The chromosome damage resulting from two years of moderate marijuana use (calculated from Stenchever's findings) is comparable in type and frequency to the chromosome damage resulting from exposure to 150 roentgens of radiation. In animal studies, interference with DNA metabolism, delayed cell division, mutations, broken chromosomes, abnormal chromosome numbers, and malformed embryos have been found to be the effects of exposure to radiation. With the exception of mutations, these effects have been observed in laboratory animals exposed to THC. (Mutation studies are now in progress.) With the exception of mutations and malformed embryos, these effects have also been observed in humans exposed to THC.

Another serious implication of damage to cells is the suppression of immune response. The immune system is maintained by certain cells that carry genes able to identify foreign proteins, to remember their identity, and to generate immune bodies to combat the foreign proteins.

A diminished immune response by certain white blood cells (lymphocytes), as measured by the suppression of their ability to divide, has been found in marijuana users (Nahas *et al.*, 1974). Fifty-one people aged sixteen to thirty-five, each of whom had smoked marijuana at least once a week (four times a week on the average) for at least one year (four years average), were tested. No drug except marijuana had been used by these subjects. The control group consisted of eighty-one healthy volunteers, twenty to seventy-two years of age. Cultures of the white blood cells (T lymphocytes) of marijuana users were compared with those of nonusers. The ability of these cells to change form, a transformation associated with protein synthesis (blast transformation, the necessary stage in the production of immune bodies), was compared. It was established that the cells of marijuana users were less able to effect this transformation. The suppression was not much greater in daily users than in weekly users. The cells of people with cancer or uremic poisoning and of those who have been treated with drugs following organ transplant to suppress immune response to foreign tissues are also less capable of making this transformation.

The conclusions of this study were confirmed in another experiment performed on monkeys exposed to marijuana smoke (Nahas, in U.S. Senate Hearings, 1974). The same suppression of immune response appeared in the monkeys. Other studies on human cells have confirmed the observation (Peterson *et al.*, 1974; Gupta *et al.*, 1974).

Other immune responses, such as that of skin cells, may not be affected by marijuana. Skin cells are exposed to much less THC than are blood cells. However, white mice given THC orally reject skin grafts from black mice of another strain more slowly than do normal mice (Munson *et al.*, 1976). This indicates a suppression of the immune response.

THC appears to lower the rate of cell division by diminishing the body's capacity to synthesize DNA, RNA, and protein (Nahas *et al.*, 1974). Related effects have been confirmed in other experiments on human cells (Blevins & Regan, 1976; Huot, 1976; Leuchtenberger *et al.*, 1976; Morishima *et al.*, 1976*a*; Stefanis & Issidorides, 1976). In another study of the effects of Δ-8- and Δ-9-THC in human leukocyte cultures (Neu *et al.*, 1970), although no evidence of structural damage was found in the chromosomes, a reduction in the rate of cell division was noted.

Experiments demonstrating that THC can alter chromosome number are further evidence that the drug can disrupt cell division. Chromosomes in the lymphocytes (white blood cells) of marijuana smokers and nonsmokers were compared. In the smokers, over 30 percent of the lymphocytes contained only from five to thirty chromosomes (the normal number is forty-six). In the nonsmokers, only 10 percent of the lymphocytes contained fewer than thirty-one chromosomes (Morishima, in U.S. Senate Hearings, 1974). Similar alterations in chromosome number were found by Leuchtenberger *et al.* (1976) and Stenchever *et al.* (1976). Altered chromosome numbers are commonly found in cancer cells.

The effects of THC on human and animal cells are studied by exposing living cells to THC (in vivo) and by exposing cells to THC in a culture dish or test tube (in vitro). Some experiments on adverse effects of marijuana have been criticized because the white blood cells were tested in vitro rather than in vivo. The criticisms are invalid, for in vitro tests on the white blood cells of marijuana smokers and nonsmokers show results that are different and significant. In addition, the same abnormalities have been observed in cells exposed to THC in both in vivo and in vitro experiments. For instance, lung cells in a tissue culture exposed to marijuana smoke had the same chromosome breaks and abnormalities as the white blood cells taken from marijuana smokers (Leuchtenberger *et al.*, 1976; Morishima *et al.*, 1976*a*).

Results of in vivo and in vitro studies on the cellular effects of marijuana were presented in 1975 at an international conference held in Helsinki. These scientific reports have been compiled in *Marijuana: Chemistry, Biochemistry, and Cellular Effects* (edited by Nahas *et al.*, 1976). Photographic evidence of marked cellular changes in human cells of hashish users are shown in this test (Stefanis & Issidorides). Photomicrographs of white blood cells show a deficiency of phospholipids in the outer cell membrane, a deficiency in basic proteins in the cell nucleus, and changes in the cell surface. Electron micrographs of sperm show that the head of the sperm contains little of the normally abundant arginine-rich protein – an indication of interruption in the final stages of protein synthesis.

The effects of marijuana on cell functions – immune response, synthesis of DNA and RNA, and protein synthesis – are probably caused by the accumulation of THC on the outer membrane surfaces of cells. THC probably also accumulates on the inner membrane surfaces, since these parts of the cell are composed of fats. Cell surfaces have concentrations of THC several hundred times greater than the blood plasma (Paton, in U.S. Senate Hearings, 1974). Inner cell membranes are important to such cell activities as synthesis of proteins of DNA from DNA and of RNA from DNA. The delay in cell division is believed to be caused by a slowing of the synthesis of DNA and proteins that are necessary for cell duplication. DNA and RNA control the synthesis of the immune proteins (antibodies) in the white blood cells (T lymphocytes).

Chromosome breakage and suppression of lymphocyte

immunity associated with marijuana use seem only slightly related to dose; nearly as much change occurs with light use as with heavy exposure. These findings suggest that the primary difficulty may be in the saturation of the cell surfaces with THC. Owing to the retention of THC, about as much THC accumulates on cell surfaces with occasional as with daily use of marijuana. The duration of use rather than the dose is the most important factor in chromosome breakage and suppression of the immune response; and, as Nahas (1975*b*) has pointed out, "one may well ask what will happen to [marijuana smokers] in a decade or two, when the aging process has further decreased their immune mechanisms." Certainly the susceptibility to infectious disease has been noted in older populations of countries where marijuana use is endemic.

Evidence for the effects of THC on DNA, RNA, the immune system, and on chromosomes is subtle. Laborious hours of careful work by highly trained experts working under controlled laboratory conditions are needed to determine such changes. Specialists in chromosome and genetic work have just begun to study populations where cannabis drugs have been used for centuries.

Effect on pregnancy and offspring

Animal experiments have shown that marijuana affects pregnancy and offspring. Although the observations of such effects on humans have not been sufficient to resolve the question, enough has been proved about the effects of marijuana on the endocrine and cell systems to suggest that the drug has an effect on pregnancy and offspring. THC administered to pregnant mice was found to accumulate in the placenta and embryonic tissue. In the group of experimental animals, the number of liveborn babies, the size of litters, and the size of the offspring all declined (Harbison & Mantilla-Plata, 1972). It has been established in three species of animals that crude cannabis administered during pregnancy causes fetal death or fetal abnormality and that these effects are dose related (Paton, in U.S. Senate Hearings, 1974). The doses used in these animal studies were high, but the results should not therefore be discounted.

Toxic substances may affect just the persons exposed (including fetuses or nursing babies of pregnant women or lactating mothers exposed to toxic substances), or, if mutagenic as well, there is a risk of altering the genes in sperm or eggs so as to have a potential effect on future generations. Marijuana has been found to alter sperm cells. Two mouse studies showed a reduction in DNA content of cells destined to become sperm (spermatids) from exposure to marijuana smoke and one showed degenerating forms of spermatids and fragmented sperm from exposure to THC (reported by Leuchtenberger *et al.*, 1976). (As discussed above, DNA is the chemical substance of genes; its structure contains the genetic code.) Electron micrographs of sperm from chronic hashish users showed consistent defective structure of the sperm due to an impairment of protein synthesis (Stefanis and Issidorides, 1976). What effects such alterations in sperm have on pregnancy and offspring have not been determined since we do not yet know the effect of marijuana on the genes themselves.

Genetic damage is usually subtle and may be recognizable only later. If exposure to a mutagenic substance continues, there is the potential for each successive generation to add damaged genes to the gene pool. The extent of the damage may be observable only as a slow decline in physical and mental vigor in future generations. "Habitual, chronic marijuana smoking," one researcher stated, "can be said to be genetic roulette" (Nahas, 1976).

Further research is needed on the effects of marijuana on

conception, fetal development, and quality of offspring. Carefully controlled studies of at least one generation and many thousands of people will be necessary to establish whether marijuana causes mutations and malformations.

Relation of animal and human studies

I have limited this discussion mainly to the effects of the cannabis drugs in human studies and have cited only a few of the key supplementary animal studies. This was done because we are concerned about the effects in humans and because the average person is not prepared to understand animal studies in drug research and is somewhat reluctant to apply the results of animal studies to humans. However, since THC was isolated, hundreds of experiments have been done showing the harmful effects of THC on animals. This work is of great importance, for it both confirms what can be observed and provides studies not possible using human subjects. The amounts of THC can be highly controlled; researchers can be sure that the animals have had no other drug except the one administered; live animals can be kept in controlled environments for careful observation; and animals can be sacrificed to examine tissue, organs, and cells. Also, genetic effects can be studied in a short span of time. Mice and rats, for example, produce litters of about ten pups and a new generation is possible three times a year. Using mice or rats, a study of the effects of a drug on the functions of organ systems and on growth and development for the entire life of the animal can be completed in three to four years.

When extending data on drug effects from animal studies to apply to humans, adjustments must be made for the differences in body size and metabolic rate. In studies of the immediate short-term effects (within, for example, about an hour after exposure), effects are related to the concentration of the drug in the blood and the major body organs. For this purpose, in comparisons between species, concentration of the drug in the blood is based on dose per kilogram of body weight. In studies of long-term effects, the duration of exposure of the major body organs becomes the main consideration. Duration of exposure is related to retention of the drug in the blood and major body organs, which is inversely proportional to the metabolic rate of the species. Metabolic rate is the energy production per unit of body weight. The metabolic rate is about three times higher in the monkey than in man, and about seven times higher in small laboratory rodents than in man. Therefore, to study the long-term effects of THC the dose administered to a monkey would have to be about three times as great as an equivalent dose for a man; the dose administered to a mouse would have to be about seven times as great. A dose of THC adjusted for metabolic rate to give equivalent long-term exposures to two species of animals will not give equivalent short-term exposures. In animals smaller than humans, the effects for about the first hour will relate to higher concentration of the THC in the blood – the consequence of giving a larger dose per unit of body weight.

In experiments on animals, substances suspected of being toxic are often administered in doses higher than the calculated equivalent for humans in order to amplify effects that might escape detection at lower doses. Also, the effects of low doses may not be observable until after long exposure. When the effects of high doses are established, the effects of lower doses are more easily identified and investigated; if significant effects occur with high doses, similar or related reduced effects are likely to be present with lower doses.

Not all animal data are applicable to humans, but most are. An animal species is often selected for research because of its similarity to human systems, and then, as discussed above, appropriate calculations are made to adjust for the differences in body size and/or metabolic rate. When several species of selected animals all react similarly, the results are usually considered highly significant for human applications.

To say, therefore, that certain drug effects have appeared only in animal studies is not to say that the same effects would not appear in humans if humans could be subjected to similar experiments. Many drugs have been banned for human use on the strength of animal experiments alone.

Because their brains are not as highly developed, animals are not as useful for studying changes in the higher cognitive functions. Behavioral changes in animals, however, have been noted to be produced by a number of sensual drugs, and the general pattern is much the same as in humans. Some cause-and-effect relationships are not measurable, such as in certain human brain functions. In studies of these relationships, the greater the number of human studies that show the same pattern of cause and effect, the more likely it is that the results will be scientifically significant. A drug should not be considered harmless because techniques are not available for measuring its effects in the laboratory.

How much marijuana is harmful?

This is a difficult question to answer because the effects of marijuana are somewhat unpredictable and highly individual. I have found that approximately one out of ten young marijuana users is extremely sensitive to the drug. This person may have residual symptoms – difficulty focusing his eyes, conversation lags, and a reduced attention span – for as long as a week after smoking a very small amount of marijuana. Other individuals are highly tolerant to marijuana. Some people have rare enzyme systems that can degrade marijuana metabolically.

Most marijuana users are between these two extremes. Certainly, anyone who smokes marijuana on a daily basis shows obvious signs of use. Although the effects on the brain from small amounts are difficult to measure by existing methods, some symptoms are undoubtedly present in all regular marijuana users. However, since many occasional users are not visibly affected, the harmfulness of marijuana is underestimated.

As we have seen, long-term use and high doses can cause irreversible changes in and outside the brain. On the other hand, recent evidence indicates that the duration of use rather than the size of the dose determines the degree of chromosome damage and suppression of the immune system. Thus the answer to the question, How much marijuana is harmful? is open, and depends on the effects one is considering.

Looking at what might be called moderate, typical use, researchers have found that marijuana has enduring, debilitating effects:

Regular users, that is, once or twice weekly, show clinical evidence of continuing low-grade intoxication, characterized by memory impairment, mood swings, sleep disturbances, and generally lessened functioning. They also show a variety of physical disorders. Both the psychological and physical symptoms usually, though not always, begin to clear up a week or two after discontinuation of cannabis use. [Schwarz, in U.S. Senate Hearings, 1974]

Kolansky and Moore (1975) studied the psychological, toxic effects of marijuana between intoxication periods in fifty-one people who smoked marijuana three or more times a week for many months. They found:

All subjects clearly demonstrated an early diminution in self-awareness and judgment along with slowed thinking and shorter spans in concentration and attention. We also reported a gradual development of "goal-lessness," blunted emotions, a counterfeit impression of calm and well-being, and a prevailing illusion of recently developed insight and emotional maturity. Many demonstrated difficulty in depth perception and an alteration in the sense of timing, both of which are particularly hazardous during automobile driving. [Kolansky & Moore, 1975]

The symptoms in all the subjects began with marijuana use and disappeared within three to twenty-four months after cessation of drug use. The symptoms corresponded to the duration and frequency of smoking. In an earlier study on the same subject, the recovery of subjects who had smoked marijuana for more than three years was incomplete (Kolansky & Moore, 1972*b*).

How is marijuana use related to multiple drug use?

My surveys of college males and the army's studies of servicemen showed that about one-half of the marijuana users took no other illicit drug (except hashish). This half generally had used marijuana infrequently for a relatively short time. As the period of marijuana use increased, the frequency of use and the dose increased, and the more likely it became that the individual would use other sensual drugs as well. A report by the Secretary of Health, Education, and Welfare (1974) has stated that "marihuana users as compared to nonusers are more likely to use or have used other, both licit and illicit, psychoactive drugs. The more heavily a user smokes marihuana, the greater the probability he has used or will use other drugs."

Most of the marijuana users I interviewed said that their use of LSD, the opiates, and cocaine followed their marijuana use. In an earlier survey in 1971, I found that 280 out of 400 college men regularly smoked marijuana; of these, 40 percent (118) had used heroin or one of the other opiates one or more times. Of the 400, 120 had not used marijuana; of the 120, none had tried opiates. In another study of 367 heroin addicts in the United States, I found that only 4 had not used marijuana before they started using heroin. In drug studies in Egypt, Soueif (1971) found that "cannabis takers far exceeded non-takers as regards attachment to alcohol, coffee, tea, and tobacco – and that they, in fact, did so before taking cannabis. However, the longer they go on taking the drug and/or the heavier they become as habitués, the more liable to adding opium to their drug menu they turn." (My survey also showed a higher percentage of marijuana smokers used tea, coffee, alcohol, and tobacco than nonsmokers; Table 9.) In another study, Soueif (1976a) found that individuals who used cannabis at least thirty times a month rarely were able to stop. If they tried to stop, they usually started using another drug in addition to cannabis. Still another survey of college students disclosed that 100 percent of the heavy marijuana

Table 9. *Relation between marijuana use and multiple drug use among college males*

Drug	1975 (spring)		1976 (spring)	
	Marijuana users[a] using drug (% of 71)	Nonusers using drug (% of 29)	Marijuana users[a] using drug (% of 79)	Nonusers using drug (% of 19)
Tea	73	55	70	63
Coffee	87	38	71	58
Alcohol	85	64	91	37
Tobacco cigarettes	41	3	35	10
Hashish	77	0	85	0
Amphetamines	49	0	52	0
LSD	58	7[b]	51	0
Cocaine	48	0	44	0
Opiates	27	0	24	0
Barbiturates	31[c]	0	20[c]	0
Tranquilizers	41[c]	7[b,c]	28[c]	0

[a] Average use: 3.2 times per week.
[b] Were former marijuana users.
[c] Includes prescribed medications.

users, 84 percent of the weekly users, and 22 percent of the monthly users had tried other drugs (Brill *et al.*, 1970).

The results of my survey of college men indicated that amphetamines and marijuana were used together more often than were barbiturates and marijuana, and that marijuana users also used tranquilizers generously. Tranquilizers were used for their calming effect rather than in high doses for their sensual effect, and thus were listed by the subjects under "medical use." Some considered barbiturates to be for medical purposes. Interestingly, marijuana users who also took tranquilizers also used more barbiturates than did other marijuana smokers. Those who used hashish started to do so following their use of marijuana. Nonusers of marijuana, even though they used alcohol, did not use illicit drugs; in my 1975 sample, two former marijuana users (7 percent) had used LSD and two had used tranquilizers (Table 9). Thus, the evidence suggests that marijuana conditions the user to the other sensual drugs.

There are several explanations of why marijuana smokers escalate to other, more sensually powerful drugs. Once a person uses a drug, he becomes involved in a drug-oriented environment. In such an atmosphere, where many kinds of drugs are available, peer pressure can be very strong. Because his powers of judgment and will are reduced, the marijuana user is highly susceptible to the enticing possibility of greater pleasure. He may also come to prefer the variety of sensations multiple drug use produces. Many multiple drug users have said in interviews that, after finding they liked marijuana, they set out to try as many other kinds of drugs as possible. A more powerful drug can also mask the restlessness, sleeplessness, and agitation of withdrawal from marijuana. Heroin, cocaine, and amphetamines, for example, hide these symptoms as well as relieve the depressed sensual response associated with tolerance to marijuana.

Most experiments and research conducted on cannabis in recent years have not considered the fact that cannabis is usually not consumed in isolation from other drugs (Tennant, in U.S. Senate Hearings, 1974). We need more research on the effects of simultaneous use of marijuana and other drugs, particularly alcohol. Alcohol consumption among drug users is increasing at a rapid rate; one survey of college students (Klein *et al.*, 1971) indicated that alcohol use by marijuana smokers is twice that of the nonsmokers. My survey showed that many more marijuana smokers used alcohol than nonsmokers (Table 9). My observations and interviews have also suggested that college marijuana users drink – especially beer and wine – for the compounding effect. As discussed in Chapter 5, marijuana users are able rapidly to increase their alcohol consumption.

The dangers are also compounded by multiple drug use. For example, marijuana can intensify and prolong the effects of barbiturates and other drugs used in medical treatment. This means that a nonlethal dose of a barbiturate could be lethal (Paton, in U.S. Senate Hearings, 1974).

Isn't marijuana the least harmful drug?

In the past, people who cautioned against the use of marijuana highly exaggerated the effects of the drug. They generated the fear, for example, that a few marijuana cigarettes could lead to prolonged insanity or violent crime. The exaggerations created much distrust when the effects experienced by marijuana smokers were not what the threats described. The trouble, however, is that when marijuana users experience no overtly debilitating effects from short-term use, they ignore all information about the harmfulness of long-term marijuana use. They like the pleasant effects and ignore or cannot recognize the drug's subtle damage. They declare that marijuana is a harmless drug. Marijuana smokers generally do not publicize their bad experiences; probably only a fraction of the serious psychic episodes caused by marijuana, for example, come to the attention of doctors. However, now that the long-term effects of marijuana use are becoming evident and scientific studies are becoming public knowledge, users and nonusers are beginning to realize that marijuana is not a safe drug.

I believe we should look upon marijuana as the most potentially dangerous of the sensuous drugs. We know now that its effects are deleterious, but insidious and subtle. Even so, the full extent of its harmfulness is probably yet to be learned. The principal dangers of marijuana use (other than the effects on the genes and the cell systems, which have already been discussed) are summarized below:

1. Unlike the other sensual drugs, marijuana's effects are usually not experienced the first few times a user takes it. Then for a time, a very small dose produces an effect, which leads the user to believe that marijuana is indeed harmless.

2. Because of the mildness of early withdrawal symptoms (as compared with those from other sensual drugs), the user thinks he is taking a mild drug and can easily withdraw any time he chooses.

3. Psychological conditioning to marijuana, in comparison with the apparent lack of chemical dependency, is strong. The user is dependent on marijuana before he realizes it, and few regular or heavy users can stop without great effort.

4. The toxic substances in marijuana accumulate in the brain and the other body tissues and leave slowly. Most users do not know that most cumulative, noxious substances have long-range effects that are not evident from short-term use. Even mild use of marijuana (regular social use, for example) produces some long-lasting effects.

5. Tolerance to marijuana builds up rapidly so that most regular users need to progress to stronger or larger doses or to use the drug more frequently to feel the effects. What originally was a pleasant experience, in time is repeated only to avoid feeling bad. The majority of marijuana users do not stay with the occasional smoking of a mild marijuana cigarette.

6. The mechanisms in the brain that the user needs to evaluate his situation are disturbed by marijuana. The user, even when he is severely

affected, cannot understand his problem.

7. For various reasons, many marijuana users tend to become heavy smokers of tobacco, to use alcohol excessively, and to go on to use stronger drugs. The effects from a combination of drugs are compounded, not simply the sum of the effects of each.

8. Marijuana use has spread in epidemic proportions among the young, who have the most to lose from it. Marijuana can retard emotional development at a crucial time in the maturing process. The adolescent is especially vulnerable, as he is developing new habits and ideas and integrating his personality into his surroundings. Sensual drugs alter body functions normally controlled by hormones. Now we know that hormone production is disturbed by marijuana. Sex hormones, delicately balanced in the adult, are in a state of flux in the adolescent.

Kolansky and Moore (1972*a*) found that "marijuana greatly accentuates the inconsistencies of behavior, the lack of control of impulses, the vagueness of thinking, and the uncertainty of body identity," so typical of adolescents. Marijuana diminishes the ability to concentrate, to motivate oneself, and to work toward goals. Soueif (1976*b*) administered tests of psychomotor speed, perception of distance and time, memory, and visual motor coordination to 850 male users of cannabis and to 839 nonusers. The performances of the younger cannabis users (below twenty-five years of age) were more significantly impaired than the performances of older users (thirty-five to fifty years of age). Lehmann (1971), director of VITAM, a drug rehabilitation foundation in Connecticut, has said: "I think that the worst thing about marijuana is that it infuses a terrible apathy into youngsters at precisely that time when they should be making or preparing to make important decisions that will affect the rest of their lives."

Perhaps those best able to give an informed account of marijuana's effects are former users themselves. I say former because only those who have stopped using drugs have a perspective on their drugged condition. Former drug users are rarely fooled by arguments for the benefits of marijuana. From these former users we can get a full story about the effects of marijuana on their lives. One told me his story:

The first few months in Berkeley I began smoking dope more and more. I remember thinking each time as I was about to get stoned that after I had a few hits and was high I would be happy. Once I was high I would find myself trapped in this labyrinth of interconnected, circular, and futile thoughts usually concerning myself, my identity, and what I was doing and what I wanted – which I was having difficulty arriving at. Then I would think to myself that being stoned wasn't making me any happier or helping me solve my problems; it was just weighing me down. Then I would tell myself I was never going to get stoned anymore, and I would remember that I had made that same resolution the last time I had been stoned. Each time I would forget the resolution before getting stoned and each time I would make it again.

Eventually I realized that I had to stop and get myself together. I realized that smoking dope was sapping my will and my energy. I had little desire to do anything other than sit around. I felt perpetually tired and everything I did attempt to do took great effort. This became extremely distasteful to me. I began disliking the whole pot party scene. People sat around stoned, each in their own worlds, not really communicating. They seemed empty and lifeless, just as I felt. After I stopped smoking dope for about a month, I felt this great, dull weight that had descended on my mind lifting. [Personal files, 1970]

Because of the subtle and insidious effects of marijuana, young and old alike are caught up without realizing the consequences. The following letter from a housewife to Ann Landers gives still another picture of the life of a marijuana user:

Dear Ann Landers:
I've seen many letters in your column from teen-agers who smoke pot, but I don't recall ever having seen a letter from a pot-smoking housewife. There must be thousands, Ann, but maybe they don't write. I might be the first.

Our four children are between the ages of three and ten. My husband and I are in the middle-income bracket – perhaps higher. We live in the suburbs and he makes about $20,000 a year. I started to smoke pot after our last baby was born. At first it relaxed me. It seemed as if I were looking at the world through rose-colored glasses. I was sure pot was the greatest thing since sliced bread. It minimized my problems and helped me cope with my children.

My husband didn't approve of pot but he never ordered me to quit using it. I should tell you I bought the stuff from a neighbor for $10 a lid. She said she started to smoke to get off booze. (Incidentally, the poor girl appears stoned most of the time and people think she still drinks.)

About six months ago my husband told me I was beginning to behave like my neighbor. I have to admit I staggered around a lot and my memory konked out. But worst of all, I was unsure of myself behind the wheel of a car. My perception of distance and time was distorted and I tried to fake it. Finally, after I had a minor accident, my husband laid down the law – NO MORE POT.

I haven't touched a joint in six months but I am still not back to normal. I get headaches (which I never had before) and I feel slightly detached. But I'm determined to become my old self again and face life's problems with whatever inner resources I can muster. No more copping out. Please print this for all my sisters who are where I was seven months ago. [Landers, 1973]

Because of the controversy over the harmfulness of marijuana, few people in responsible positions – civic leaders, lawyers, doctors, or parents – are willing to take a stand against marijuana, thus leaving the younger generation without authorities or models to follow. For example, a recent study showed that 80 percent of the medical students surveyed used marijuana. It is to be hoped that when medical students understand the dangers of marijuana use, they will stop using it, just as doctors stopped smoking when it was discovered that tobacco smoking had serious, harmful consequences. Twenty years ago, 70 percent of physicians smoked; today it is estimated that only about 7 percent have continued the habit.

Americans are now consuming far greater quantities of cannabis and far stronger preparations of cannabis than they were a few years ago (see Appendix 10 and U.S. Senate Hearings, 1975). Seizures of hashish by United States authorities have escalated from over 7,000 pounds in 1970 to over 50,000 pounds in 1973–1974. Hashish oil, which had never appeared in significant amounts on the illicit market in America, now turns up more frequently. In 1974, 369 pounds was seized. The THC content of hashish ranges from almost none in old samples to as much as 20 percent in fresh, high-grade samples. Middle Eastern hashish is about 10 percent THC; hashish oil is from 20 to 90 percent THC.

According to estimates made from the marijuana seized by American authorities, the quantity of marijuana consumed in the United States has doubled each year from 1969 through 1974. The potency of bulk marijuana seized in the United States has increased from less than 1 percent THC before 1970 to about 1 percent in 1970 and to 3 to 4 percent in 1975–1976. The THC content of some seizures has been reported to be as high as 14 percent. High potency marijuana comes from tropical sources; in the street trade, it is usually blended with domestic marijuana, but some is sold as premium grade at high prices. Thus, although marijuana cigarettes sold on the streets today are usually 1 to 3 percent THC, the THC content may be as high as 14 percent.

Are marijuana and alcohol comparable?

Alcoholism is now considered the fourth major health problem in the United States (Klein *et al.*, 1971), but many people still say that because alcohol is legal, marijuana should be too. The arguments equate alcohol with marijuana, but the fact is that the two drugs are *not* equivalent and should not be treated so.

The major difference is that marijuana's principal active ingredient is highly soluble in fat and insoluble in water; THC remains in the fat structures of the cells for long periods and, with repeated use, accumulates there. Alcohol, on the other hand, is a water-soluble food and is therefore metabolized to provide cell energy. It leaves the body very rapidly and completely; there is no residue. Also, molecule for molecule, THC is 10,000 times stronger than alcohol in its ability to produce mild intoxication, and small amounts of marijuana linger as much as 10,000 times longer in the body. For example, one drink containing 10 grams of ethyl alcohol is metabolized into carbon dioxide, water, and acetone in an average-sized person in about one hour; 50 grams of alcohol produces mild intoxication and is metabolized in about five hours. Only 5 milligrams (0.005 gram) of THC absorbed into the body produces the same degree of intoxication. At the end of one week, 30 percent is still in the body; at the end of seven weeks, 10 percent remains. Repeated use adds more. Even after marijuana use is completely stopped, it takes months for all the THC to leave the body. The marijuana user is under the influence of the drug even between highs.

In addition, marijuana, like opium, is a complex mixture of dozens of chemical constituents, each of which may have very different effects on the body. Some chemical and pharmacological features of the cannabinoids are, in fact, more similar to those of the opiates than of alcohol. The effects of marijuana are different from alcohol in many ways. THC damages chromosomes; alcohol does not. THC affects DNA,RNA, and the immune response; alcohol does not. Irreversible brain changes are apparent after only three years of daily marijuana use; it takes decades for irreversible brain changes to appear in the heavy drinker. Three people in six who use marijuana are likely to become addicted; one person in six who uses alcohol is likely to become addicted.

Making a comparison between alcohol and cannabis, one researcher said: "The price [in health] for its [cannabis] overuse is paid in adolescence or in early life; . . . the price . . . for alcohol overuse is paid in later life" (Paton, in

U.S. Senate Hearings, 1974). One other difference between the drugs is that marijuana intoxication is more difficult to detect than drunkenness. Those under the influence of alcohol show definite, outward signs of their condition, and simple legal tests exist for determining the alcohol content of the breath, blood, and urine. A simple, practical test for detecting THC residue on the lips and fingers has been developed. Marijuana can be detected up to six hours after it is taken, depending on the strength of the marijuana and how it was smoked (Kier, 1975). Although research is being done to find a way of detecting marijuana in the body, at this time there is no practical, accurate test. For the operation of any machinery, especially automobiles or airplanes, this raises questions of both safety and legality.

Marijuana is becoming one of the major problem drugs. Out of 41,873 admissions to federally financed treatment clinics (see Chapter 5), marijuana was given as the reason for admission two and one-half times more often than was alcohol. In fact, marijuana ranked above alcohol and next to opiates both in the number of people admitted who used the drug and in the number who gave it as the main reason for seeking treatment.

What about the evidence that marijuana is harmless?

Many widely publicized studies have examined the effects of marijuana. Because of the nature of the research and the number of variables involved, the results of these studies have often seemed inconsistent or contradictory. Frequently reviewers who do not know how to deal with the variables evaluate the reports inaccurately, and sometimes the public is led to believe that the reports are proof that marijuana is a harmless drug.

The variables make evidence hard to evaluate. Until Δ-9-THC was isolated and measured quantities could be used, the strength of marijuana used in experiments could not be controlled. We know now that many studies that "proved marijuana was harmless" used amounts of THC that were too small to be effective. Even now, because of the nature of many studies, researchers must rely on marijuana with an unknown THC content bought on the street. Interpretations of what constitutes "light" and "heavy" use vary: some investigators define heavy use as five to ten joints per week; others, as five to ten joints per day. The amount of THC actually absorbed by an individual cannot be measured easily, and THC is not the only active ingredient in marijuana. Furthermore, over months of time marijuana declines in potency; to be certain of the THC content in the marijuana used, it needs to be assayed for THC content at the time of use.

The way the drug is taken (by smoking, injecting, or eating it), the psychological and physical condition of the user, and the length of time of exposure to THC are other variables. Also, accurate interpretation is difficult because investigators must rely on the subject's own account of his drug use. Even if the subject is truthful, his evaluation is still subjective. Whether a subject is a user or nonuser affects the conclusions. First-time users seldom feel any effect; experienced users have probably built up a tolerance, but at some stages of their use, they may need only small amounts of THC to get an effect. Also, many studies concerned with short-term effects were quoted as evidence for the harmlessness of marijuana; the conclusions were premature, for it has now been demonstrated that marijuana has harmful long-term effects. Finally, laboratory techniques can vary tremendously; it often requires someone skilled in the interpretation of scientific data to evaluate the results of a study.

In evaluating the conclusions drawn from any marijuana study, several questions must be asked: What are the variables in the study? Are the conclusions drawn from the data appropriate? How should the conclusions be qualified?

I have analyzed two studies concluding that marijuana use does not affect motivation or scholastic performance. One of the studies, performed in 1970 and 1973 on the campus where I teach (Mellinger *et al.*, 1976), analyzed the relationship between drug use and motivation. In the study, the amotivated student was identified as one who ultimately dropped out of the university. In a general sample of 834 students, 3 percent of the students who had never used marijuana dropped out, 6 percent of the students who had used only marijuana dropped out, and 14 percent of the students who used marijuana more extensively (along with other drugs) dropped out. Then a subsample of 516 of the most highly motivated students was observed. In the subsample, family background, relationship with parents, achievement in high school, and other sociocultural factors were used as predictors of motivation for users and nonusers. In this subsample, the researchers reported that there was no difference in the dropout rate (2 percent) of marijuana users and nonusers. The researchers concluded that sociocultural factors rather than marijuana use therefore caused students to leave school.

A closer look at the data, however, reveals that in selecting the group of the most highly motivated students from the general sample, the researchers necessarily eliminated a number of the heavier drug users. The number of students in the general sample and the subsample in each of the three categories of drug use are in Table 10. From these figures, it can be seen that the reduction in dropout rate is the result of the elimination of the heavier marijuana users from the subsample, for the adjustment itself shows that there is a correlation between achievement and drug use.

Further analysis of this study shows that the students in the general sample who used marijuana were light users –70

Table 10. *Effect of subsample selection on findings regarding relation of marijuana use to motivation*

Drug use	General sample (no.)	Highly motivated students (no.)	Students eliminated from general sample to make up subsample (%)
Never smoked marijuana	344	278	19
Used only marijuana	302	183	39
Used marijuana more extensively and used other drugs	188	55	71

percent averaged only two days of use a month. The selection of the subsample, which eliminated the heavier marijuana users, resulted in a sample of the very light users. When the average use was so light, it is not surprising that the researchers found factors other than marijuana use caused students to drop out.

In another study of marijuana users in a university population, Brill and Christie (1974) concluded that there were no significant differences between the grade point averages and educational achievement of users and nonusers. In analyzing their data I find that to make these conclusions they treated the marijuana-using students as a group, 70 percent of whom smoked marijuana only an average of two times per month. They did not examine separately the records of the 11 percent of the marijuana-smoking students who were regular users. Also, the quantity and grade of marijuana were not considered in the study. The marijuana used was probably mild, as potent marijuana was not generally available on college campuses in the early 1970s. To determine accurately the effect of marijuana on student achievement studies should be conducted that consider the degree of exposure to THC. The potency of the marijuana used, the frequency of use, and the amount used at any one time all need to be considered.

It should be noted in evaluating such studies that grades and dropout rate may not be sensitive measures of the effects of marijuana on academic achievement. I have observed that students often reduce their course loads and transfer from difficult to easier courses of study before their grades drop and before they drop out of school. This tendency keeps grade point averages higher and the dropout rates lower than they might otherwise be.

The findings of one study cannot be used as evidence to disprove the findings of another unless the significant variables in each investigation are comparable. For example, the studies done to date that show no increase in chromosome breakage from marijuana cannot be used to disprove the observation of Stenchever *et al.* (1974) that the white cells of marijuana users had a significant increase in chromosome breakage. These studies differed from Stenchever's in significant ways such as using short-term exposures to marijuana, controls who had been exposed to marijuana previously, and different laboratory techniques. Also, the oral ingestion rather than smoking of marijuana may have made a difference since, as discussed above, high temperatures convert some of the inactive cannabinols to THC.

The following two studies are given as other examples of the necessity to examine the data and techniques carefully before making comparisons between studies. As discussed above, Nahas *et al.* (1974) reported that chronic marijuana smokers showed a decrease of cell-mediated immune response. Lau *et al.* (1976) reported the results of a study intended to check these findings by eliminating uncertainty about the dose of Δ-9-THC through the use of orally administered measured doses. Lau's results appear to show no effect of Δ-9-THC on immunity. Close examination of these two studies suggests, however, that the latter cannot serve as a check of the former.

Nahas used sufficiently large groups of subjects (eighty-one controls, fifty-one marijuana smokers) and controlled techniques to achieve consistent readings of the synthesis of DNA in lymphocytes after challenges with each of two agents. His standard errors when cells were tested with PHA (the agent, phytohemagglutinin) were 0.9 percent for the controls and 1.2 percent for the smokers, corresponding to standard deviations of 6.8 percent and 18.3 percent, respectively. In comparing smokers and controls, he found a significant difference of 41 percent.

Lau, on the other hand, used only eight smokers and eight controls in one trial and seven smokers in another, with an unreported but undoubtedly small number of controls, in view of the large standard deviation reported. For example, at the lowest PHA dosage, the range corresponding to ±1 standard deviation for the controls tested by Lau, as read from her graph (no data are tabulated), is about 115 to 2,600 counts per minute. Compare the ±1 standard deviation range for Nahas's controls: approximately 21,350 to 25,150 counts per minute. The variability in Lau's results would easily obscure the extent of change observed by Nahas. Many differences in technique could account for this discrepancy in observations. For example, Nahas began his tests immediately on freshly drawn blood samples. Lau began her tests on unrefrigerated blood samples after variable time lags up to twenty-four hours.

It would be impossible to evaluate here all the marijuana studies that have been done. However, there are, in particular, five reports done by various governments that are most often quoted as evidence that marijuana is a harmless drug. The conclusions of these reports are widely circulated, but the qualifying factors, the failures to look closely at the evidence, are rarely, if ever, noted. A discussion of each of these reports follows, and the results of two very recent studies are also noted.

Indian Hemp Drugs Commission Report (1894)

This was the first attempt to evaluate the effects of cannabis drug use on a population. Throughout the 1960s, this report was cited to support the claim that marijuana is a mild intoxicant.

The study was done in India by a commission appointed by the British government. It involved 1,140 witnesses who were given seventy questions to answer orally or in writing. Most of the conclusions were based on the collection of 1,140 conflicting opinions. There were many problems with the report:

The undertaking of the Indian Hemp Drugs Commission was . . . doomed from the beginning to report ambiguous results. . . . As the commissioners themselves pointed out, it was impossible to obtain proper records, accurate statistics, or reliable information since many of the subjects under investigation were illiterate peasants. It was impossible to dissociate the effects of hemp drugs per se from those of all the other "vices in which a dissipated man indulges." It was a "can of worms." But instead of acknowledging the impossibility, under such muddled circumstances, of establishing a cause-effect relationship between hemp drugs and physical or mental effects, they gave cannabis the benefit of the doubt. . . .

They acknowleged that excessive use of hemp was harmful but that moderate use was not. However, they failed to define what they meant by moderate and excessive, both in terms of quantity or material used and of frequency of use. [Nahas, 1973]

A report of dissenting views that presented evidence for the harmful effects of cannabis was appended to the commission's report. Even in the main body of the report, witnesses noted harmful effects besides the evidence gathered by the commission that linked mental illness with cannabis use. From information gathered from mental asylums in India, the commission found that about 18 percent of the patients were hemp users; 7.3 percent of the illnesses were attributed to hemp drug effects, and 11.6 percent were diagnosed as due to the use of hemp drugs. This was a significant discovery since, in the general population, hemp users constituted only about 0.6 percent. The dissenting opinion stated that hemp drugs were a significant cause of mental illness in India.

It is interesting to note that the damage to the lungs, brain, and liver; suppressed semen production; intestinal disturbances; and general debilitation of health from cannabis use reported by witnesses in the 1894 Indian Hemp Drugs Commission Report are now being substantiated scientifically.

When evaluating the conclusions of the India Report, one must consider that at that time, hemp was a major crop in India, that cannabis drug use was legal, and that it was used medically and in some religious ceremonies. The initial instruction issued to the commission by a government official warned that "restrictive measures of a stringent character may give rise to a serious discontent and be resented by the people as an unjustified interference with long-established social customs." Also, the commission's conclusions on the harmlessness of cannabis were based not so much on the effects of cannabis on an individual as on the fact that the commission did not consider the 0.6 percent incidence of cannabis use in India a serious enough problem in 1894 to warrant a confrontation. (It is interesting to note that the incidence of cannabis drug use in the United States in 1976 was about 15 percent.) The dissenting opinion, however, warned that the use of hemp drugs in India was increasing as a result of the expanding Indian hemp industry.

La Guardia Report (1944)

This report, officially titled *The Marihuana Problem in the City of New York* (New York City Mayor's Committee on Marihuana, 1944), analyzed the first large-scale study of the acute effects of marijuana done in the United States. The study was composed of two parts: a sociological investigation and clinical and pharmacological studies. The report has been eagerly accepted by many people as evidence that marijuana use does not cause permanent harm, is not addictive, and does not lead to the use of harder drugs.

The clinical study observed the effects of marijuana on volunteers, mostly prison inmates. Although the study was for the most part a comprehensive investigation, it primarily measured acute effects from mild marijuana. The report stated that when subjects were allowed to smoke as many marijuana cigarettes as they wanted, they used between two and thirteen cigarettes a day. It also said that "they all stated that the habit had often been interrupted voluntarily and the enforced discontinuance of it had caused no discomfort." These two statements indicate that the marijuana must have been quite mild. In my experience, daily users of moderately strong marijuana usually have difficulty quitting. Also indicative of the mildness of the marijuana used in the study is the report that the subjects, if they reached a state that was "too high," could counteract the effects with beer, soda pop, or a cold bath.

Of special significance is the fact that all the users were studied after they had been off marijuana for between two months and two years. Therefore, most subjects would have recovered from any long-term effects they may have felt. The users, then, were actually nonusers at the beginning of the study, eliminating the possibility of measuring chronic effects during the time of the study.

In the controlled studies, the usual range of effects was noted: reddened eyes, increased heartbeat, dryness of the throat, hunger, unsteadiness, dizziness, deleterious effects on mental functioning, euphoria, anxiety, hallucinations, and psychotic episodes. What the investigators did not know then was that these symptoms indicate brain changes whose permanence depends on dose and the duration of use.

Kalant, reviewing the La Guardia Report, stated:

The conclusion that marijuana smoking does not lead to physical or mental deterioration or to physical addiction was based primarily on an examination of 48 subjects. Ten of these were occasional users, 29 had used the drug for less than 10 years and only 9 had used it for 10 years or more. The number of subjects seems too small to permit valid conclusions in these respects. This is comparable to concluding that alcohol does not produce addiction from an examination of 48 beer drinkers. . . . The Mayor's Report, like many such investigations, is a valuable contribution to knowledge of cannabis, but its limitations in scope and design detract from its general applicability. [Kalant, 1968]

In the light of present knowledge about marijuana, different conclusions would be drawn in many cases. Stating that marijuana is not addictive, for example, the report said: "The absence of any compelling urge to use the drug, the absence of any distressing abstinence symptoms, the statements that no increase in dosage is required to repeat the desired effects in users – justifies the conclusion that neither true addiction nor tolerance is found in marijuana users."

The fact is, the report gave evidence that doses were increased to bring about desired effects, indicating that a degree of tolerance had indeed developed. We now know, too, that owing to the cumulative effects of marijuana, only a gradual increase in dose is needed to maintain sensual effects, and the withdrawal symptoms are mild.

The La Guardia Report, in fact, indicated the cumulative effects without exploring the implications of the statement.

What the La Guardia Report gave as lack of evidence for tolerance and addiction, we now know describes the cumulative effects of marijuana:

There is agreement in the statements that among users the smoking of one or two cigarettes is sufficient to bring on the effect known as "high." When this state is reached, the user will not continue smoking for fear of becoming "too high." When the desired effects have passed off and the smoker has "come down" smoking one cigarette brings the "high" effect on again. [New York City Mayor's Committee on Marijuana, 1944]

Shafer Commission Report (1972)

With the rise of sensual drug abuse in the United States, Congress and President Nixon appointed the U.S. National Commission on Marihuana and Drug Abuse (the Shafer Commission) to study all aspects of marijuana use. The conclusions of the report are ambiguous: the report essentially recommended that the use of marijuana be discouraged, but it also recommended that the private use of marijuana be made legal and that public sale, use, and possession continue to be illegal. Experts have been highly critical of this committee; they have felt that some of the members were biased in favor of marijuana and rejected available information on its harmful effects.

One critic, a member of the Drug Advisory Committee in Canada, referring to both the Shafer Commission and the Le Dain Commission of Canada, testified:

Both Commissions were obviously extremely selective. They did not ask for testimony from a number of people who might have said things of a more cautionary nature. I am very familiar with that activity in Canada. I know of many people who were concerned about marijuana who were not invited to testify, and I know perfectly well there were many Americans and other people who were not asked to testify here. So there was a kind of bias initially in favor of improving the climate of acceptance of marijuana on the grounds that it was criminalization that represented the real problem and not the possibly deleterious effect of the drug itself on the general population. [Malcolm, in U.S. Senate Hearings, 1974]

Another review of the report was also critical:

The commission, in summarizing its findings, published as *Marijuana: A Signal of Misunderstanding: First Report on Marijuana and Drug Abuse*, seems to have selected the data necessary to justify its rather sanguine conclusions about the use of marijuana. In our opinion, however, the actual data, contained in the Commission's two-volume, 1,252-page appendix of technical papers, should lead to the conclusion that widespread marijuana usage would be most detrimental to the American people. [Nahas & Greenwood, 1974]

And in formulating its conclusion, the Shafer Commission unfortunately ignored its own data regarding the hazards of marijuana:

Looking only at the effects on the individual, there is little proven danger of physical or psychological harm from the *experimental or intermittent* [italics mine] use of the natural preparations of cannabis, including the resinous mixtures commonly used in this country. . . . Prolonged duration of use does increase the probability of some behavioral and organic consequences including the possible shift to a heavy use pattern. The heavy users show strong psychological dependence on marijuana and often hashish. Organ injury, especially diminution of pulmonary function, is possible. Specific behavioral changes are detectable. [U.S. National Commission on Marihuana and Drug Abuse, 1972]

These statements have confused the public. Marijuana advocates have emphasized the first part and ignored the second. Unless a person has read the report, he is likely to be unaware of the cautionary statements it contained. One member of the commission testified before a congressional committee:

The Commission report, I thought, presented a fairly balanced picture; but what emerged from it, in the public consciousness, was quite unbalanced. . . . The negative side of this picture, the unpleasant side, had to be faced. . . . Scientific reports which have become available since the report was written confirm still further the need for caution. . . . I may add that in my view, marijuana must still be classed as a dangerous drug, dangerous to enough people to warrant full control. I don't distinguish sharply between hashish and marijuana; these are different concentrations of the same principle. [Brill, in U.S. Senate Hearings, 1974]

Furthermore, the Shafer Report concluded that, although the heavy use of marijuana was dangerous, most of the American experience was "with low doses of weak preparations of the drug." It was little publicized, however, that the conclusion that marijuana was a relatively mild drug was based on low doses of weak marijuana. Also, in comparing cannabis drug use in the United States with that in countries where these drugs have been used heavily for centuries, the commission stated: "At present, the Commission is unaware of any similar pattern in this country." Although the commission did recognize the dangers of heavy use, it seemed not to take seriously the fact that people in this country escalate to high doses and to stronger preparations when they are available. This has occurred in countries where cannabis drugs have been used for centuries and among American soldiers in Germany and Vietnam.

Le Dain Commission Reports (1970–1973)

Because of a growing concern over drug abuse, the Canadian government in 1969 appointed the Commission of Inquiry into the Nonmedical Use of Drugs. The Le Dain Commission, as it was commonly called, published four reports: the Interim Report (1970), the Treatment Report (1972), the Cannabis Report (1972), and the Final Report (1973). When the Interim Report appeared, it was severely criticized for its "errors and omissions," its conclusion that marijuana is a harmless drug, and its emphasis on the problems caused by its illegal status rather than on the drug itself. Many saw the report as part of a campaign to legalize the drug.

Some of the personnel who worked on the Interim Report presented special problems to the commission. One of the senior research associates who was, according to the report, "concentrating on psychopharmacological research into the effects of drugs" and who helped write the chapter, "The Drugs and Their Effects," was subsequently convicted for possession of hashish. It is reported that four other members of the supportive staff – field representatives and research assistants – were also convicted at various times for possession of hashish or marijuana. Others were reported to be users. A young professional person I happened to meet in Afghanistan in 1973, who had compiled data for the Le Dain Commission, said that it was common knowledge that many of the workers had conscientiously collected information that favored marijuana and that many of the experiments were, in his opinion, "rigged." He had come to Afghanistan to use hashish, but a severe illness resulting from his drug abuse had led him to the rehabilitation center where I met him. His abstinence and recovery had led to a change in his opinion concerning the harmlessness of marijuana.

The commission's second volume, on cannabis, subsequently presented the harmful effects of marijuana more fully and reversed the position on the mildness of the drug. It stated: "What has come to our attention with respect to long-term effects since the Interim Report is a matter for cautious concern rather than optimism."

Jamaican Report (1972)

Officially titled *The Effects of Chronic Smoking of Cannabis in Jamaica*, this study was contracted by the U.S. National Institute of Mental Health. One of the most recent studies quoted as evidence that marijuana is safe, it concluded that there are no harmful physical or mental effects from long-term use.

Although this study has been widely publicized, it has never been freely available to the general public in its complete form. The copy of the report available to the public

(U.S. Department of Health, Education, and Welfare, 1973) consists of a few paragraphs of conclusions – without the data upon which they were based. In 1975, two of the many researchers of the study, Rubin and Comitas, produced an edited version of the report. Although the editing was obviously necessary (the original report had more than 600 pages, and the edited version only 205), significant observations and conclusions were omitted in the process. For instance, two of the researchers (whose section of the report, incidentally, was the only one to appear in a scientific journal) reported the following:

No significant differences in work record could be demonstrated between smokers and nonsmokers. It may be that a difference could have been demonstrated if our sample had included intellectual workers or white-collar workers of any kind, but in a sample made up mainly of fishermen, subsistence farmers, and unskilled or partly skilled manual workers from villages where there is relatively little mobility, such differences were not detectable.

For a more complete answer to the question of the amotivational syndrome it would seem desirable to examine samples of students or other more competitive groups. [Beaubrun & Knight, 1973]

In the version of the report edited by Rubin and Comitas, only the first sentence of that section appeared.

The most publicized part of the Jamaican Report is the claim that users of ganja (potent marijuana) showed no more chromosome damage than nonusers and, in fact, showed slightly less. Because it was impossible, according to the report, to enlist enough working-class males of the right age who had never once used ganja, the control group consisted of thirty subjects, eighteen of whom had smoked ganja in the past. This, in itself, would invalidate the chromosome study, since broken chromosomes do not repair themselves no matter how much time has elapsed. In fact, the *controls* in the Jamaican study had as much chromosome breakage as the marijuana users in the Stenchever study of chromosome breakage cited earlier.

The extent of marijuana use in the "control" group in the Jamaican study is uncertain, since at least 60 percent had used marijuana at some time in the past. In addition, over half the serum samples in the study were discarded owing to faulty laboratory culture media. According to an official paper on this report:

Twenty-seven cultures from twelve users and fifteen controls failed to produce adequate results for analysis. Either there was complete failure of mitotic activity or the quality of the cells was inadequate for examination. Part of this high failure rate was due to a bad batch of calf serum used in our culture medium. It is not known without repeating the examinations whether this was the only factor. [Thorburn, 1972]

The study has also been criticized because the cells were sampled after forty-eight hours of culture and only twelve to twenty-five cells per subject were examined (Nahas, 1975*a*). Furthermore, cell cultures in the defective medium were accepted when they appeared to have some degree of mitotic activity or "reasonably normal" cell appearance. These difficulties, acknowledged by the Jamaican study, invalidate the observations. Chromosome studies require expertise and technical precision. Such inaccuracy would not be acceptable to any expert in the field of chromosome study. This may account for the fact that the study has never been published fully in a scientific journal here.

Although the authors of the Jamaican Report concluded that there were no significant changes in hormone levels from marijuana use, my analysis of their data indicates that this was not the case. Because of the small number of subjects whose urine was tested for hormone levels (seven controls and thirteen marijuana users), the difference between users and nonusers for each of the *separate* hormones tested for was not significant. However, when the results for each of the separate hormones are combined, a significant difference is evident ($P = <0.01$). Although the study did not test blood samples for changes in hormone levels, the increase in urinary elimination of steroid hormones indicates a probable lowering of the levels of these hormones in the blood.

One of the best documented parts of the Jamaican study was done on the work performance of farmers before, during, and after smoking marijuana as recorded on videotape and measured by metabolic techniques. Less work was usually accomplished per unit of time after smoking. Although the farmers themselves reported that they were doing a better job, the number of body movements per minute was usually greater, and more movements were required to complete a given task. The report said: "The extra movements per time and space unit may be related to cumulative inaccuracies, resulting in the need for repetition." This significant finding, however, was overlooked in the summary, which stated: "No significant physical or mental abnormalities could be attributed to marijuana use."

The Jamaican Report has been discredited by J. Hall, Chairman of the Department of Medicine, Kingston Hospital, Jamaica. He stated publicly:

The study does not have the general support of experienced clinicians and other workers in the field. We believe that the selection with which the study was done was faulty and that in regard to the reported absence of any change in the chromosome pattern that their technique was faulty and that certainly as regards the statement that there was no respiratory effect, it is unfounded. [Hall, in U.S. Senate Hearings, 1974]

Hall believes that the great majority of doctors in Jamaica who have had actual experience with marijuana smokers are convinced that the drug has substantial negative effect.

Brill (U.S. Senate Hearings, 1974) has also given his opinion on the findings of the report: "Finally, one should note the comment from Jamaica in the West Indies where the effects of cannabis had been thought to be relatively benign; among the middle class it is now found to be associated with school dropouts, transient psychosis, panic states, and adolescent behavior disorders."

Other reports

As this book goes to press, two other studies funded by the United States government, one in Greece and one in Costa Rica, have been quoted as new evidence that marijuana use is not harmful. Comprehensive evaluations of these studies will take time. However, considering what we know now about the dangers of marijuana use, we can probably conclude that these studies were too limited in scope to detect the damage marijuana can cause. The subjects were selected for their good health; no chromosome or related cytological studies were included, and deep brain wave analyses were not attempted. Additionally the numbers of subjects were small in comparison with the studies done by the Chopras in India and Soueif in Egypt that found harmful effects from chronic use of cannabis drugs. Using the Greek and Costa Rican studies, or the Jamaican study, as proof that marijuana is harmless is like using selected tests on a small number of healthy tobacco smokers to prove that tobacco is not detrimental to health. If more appropriate tests were used and if the group of subjects were more representative of the range of users, the harmful effects would be more apparent. Indeed, another study (Stefanis & Issidorides, 1976), which received little publicity, found basic chemical changes in the white blood cells and sperm in chronic cannabis users in Greece. It is reported to be the same group of cannabis users who had been given a nearly clean bill of health a few months earlier when examined by conventional clinical methods (Nahas, 1976).

Media misinterpretation of reports

The recent lobbying in many states to liberalize the marijuana laws has flooded the American public with conflicting statements on the harmfulness of marijuana use. The public is not prepared to distinguish among fact, misinformation, and propaganda. The average person has to rely on the evaluation of others. Unfortunately, many people who are not trained in analyzing highly specialized physiological research data, such as members of the news media, lawyers, and politicians, attempt to make these evaluations. For example, at the time of the signing of the bill decriminalizing the marijuana laws (a step essentially removing much of the legal restraint over use and possession of marijuana in California), the *San Francisco Chronicle* ran an editorial titled "Science Acquits Pot of Real Harms." It stated that "by happy coincidence, the bill was signed as the findings of an extensive study on marijuana smoking contracted by the Center for Studies of Narcotic and Drug Abuse of the National Institute of Mental Health, were made public" (*San Francisco Chronicle*, July 10, 1975). Thus, a three-year-old, much discredited work (the Jamaican Report) was cited as new sweeping evidence that Californians need not worry about the harms of marijuana smoking.

As this book goes to press, the findings of papers presented at the New York Academy of Sciences Conference on Chronic Cannabis Use are being reported by the news media. The recent study done in Costa Rica is cited as evidence that chronic use of marijuana is not associated with permanent or irreversible impairment of intelligence or higher brain function. The media have failed, however, to report another paper presented at the conference which described a major twenty-five-year study of several hundred cannabis users, sponsored by the Egyptian government, that indicates users have consistent and significant psychological function deficits (Soueif, 1976*b*). Soueif's work also provides a basis for a reevaluation of studies (such as those done in Jamaica, Greece, and Costa Rica) of older, largely illiterate subsistence farmers or unskilled workers in areas where cannabis use is endemic. Soueif has observed that mental impairment as a result of cannabis use is least apparent in these groups and that the young, literate user suffers the greatest impairment of mental functions from chronic cannabis use. None of this was mentioned by the press.

A few days after the New York Academy of Sciences conference, the fifth annual report of the U.S. Department of Health, Education, and Welfare on marijuana and health was released, and Robert L. DuPont, Director of the National Institute of Drug Abuse, held a press conference. Headlines across the country reported him as saying that tobacco and alcohol cause far greater health problems than marijuana does. What he actually said was that at current levels of use, more people have health problems from alcohol and tobacco than from marijuana. He cautioned that marijuana use is increasing, however, and that the consequences of its use may be much more serious than we now know. He also said: "There is now a very broad consensus in the United States that marijuana use should be discouraged and that the government's role is to discourage marijuana use." This statement was not mentioned in the news reports.

Is decriminalization the answer?

At the present time in the United States there are conflicting opinions concerning laws against marijuana. There is an increasing desire by a segment of the public and some legislators to have the law recognize in some way the fact that tens of millions of citizens use marijuana. Some people want marijuana completely legalized; others want to reduce penalties for possession to a citation with a fine (popularly called decriminalization). In some states, this has been done. In California, for example, marijuana laws have been liberalized to the extent that a person caught with 1 ounce or less of marijuana (enough to roll about twenty cigarettes) is given just a warning or a citation. If a citation is given, the maximum fine can be no more than $100. The record of such a citation is automatically destroyed after two years. It is no offense for a person to be under the influence of marijuana. If more than 1 ounce is confiscated and there is no intent to sell, the arresting officer has the option to either cite or arrest. In either event, the penalty can be no more than a $500 fine and/or six months in jail. Intent to sell cannot be proved by quantity alone; there must be some other evidence of selling. Under the old law, simple possession of large amounts was enough to prove intent.

As marijuana use has increased over the last decade, the enforcement of laws against the use of marijuana has decreased. We consequently have a de facto legalization of marijuana, and lawmakers are trying to adjust the law to fit the real situation. Fifty states, each responsible for legislating its own laws on marijuana control, will undoubtedly generate debate and adjustments on laws and law enforcement policies in the United States for many years.

Many recent study groups, most notably the Shafer Commission, have recommended that personal possession and use of marijuana be decriminalized and also (but with little public exposure) that marijuana use be discouraged. A few states have decriminalized their marijuana laws.

I am concerned about decriminalization for several reasons. First, much emphasis is placed on changing the laws to ease the legal problems of the marijuana user, and no emphasis is placed on warning the public about the dangers of marijuana and on discouraging its use. Second, the "shelters" in the new laws make it easy for users and pushers to circumvent the law. For the marijuana user, decriminalization essentially becomes legalization. Third, there has been no apparent concern for the international implications if the United States abandons its agreements to the United Nations Single Convention to uphold its marijuana laws.

I am concerned about the steady conversion to marijuana use of those who were previously nonusers. Warnings or mere fines for possession do little to prevent further spread. For example, in most cases, the decriminalization laws carry no more penalty for giving away marijuana than for its possession. A friend (or unidentified pusher) can easily and with very little risk (in fact, legally in one state at this time) give small amounts of marijuana to others. To avoid the risk of arrest for possession of large amounts of marijuana, small amounts may be stored in several places. Since the possession of a large quantity does not, in most cases, constitute proof of intent to sell, the risk of being arrested as a pusher is reduced.

I am concerned about further changes in the laws that will encourage marijuana use. The marijuana advocates admit decriminalization of the marijuana laws is just a step in their attempt to legalize marijuana fully. Admittedly their next goal is to throw out laws against possession altogether, to remove penalties for cultivation, and to permit marijuana to be prescribed for medical use. The advocates are attempting to shift marijuana and cannabis resin from the list of the most controlled drugs under international treaty obligations to a lesser list. And now that the movement to decriminalize marijuana has been successful in a few states, leaders of the movement are beginning to ask why it is a crime to sell marijuana if it is not a crime to possess bought marijuana.

The more widespread the use of marijuana, the easier it is to convince society of the need to soften the laws. I saw marijuana pushed on young people at the beginning of the drug movement in Berkeley. Subsequently, the use of marijuana spread. There was no obvious use of marijuana on my university campus prior to 1965, but in 1976 my sampling of male college students showed that over 75 percent had tried marijuana at least once. The Gallup surveys of drug use among college students (1967–1972) showed a steady rise in marijuana use. In 1967 only 5 percent of college students said they had tried the drug at least once; in 1969, 22 percent had used it; by 1970, 42 percent had; in 1972 the figure had climbed to 51 percent. Use of marijuana spread rapidly to high school students. Annual surveys of drug use among high school students showed those who smoked marijuana ten or more times during the previous year to be 17.5 percent in 1968, 26.3 percent in 1970, and 34.5 percent in 1972 (Blumberg, 1975). Marijuana was presented to this generation of youth as a harmless drug. Before the dangers of the drug could become known, its use spread. Now, because there are so many marijuana users, some people want to see the drug legalized.

It is true that the laws should not remain as they are. Presently, marijuana laws are different throughout the states and consequently inequitable. Nor should everyone who is apprehended for using marijuana be given a jail sentence – certainly first-time or perhaps even second-time offenders should not – nor should they incur criminal records. The law should take a clear and consistent stand, however, against the use of marijuana. To do this it must establish a definitive standard that makes clear that marijuana is a harmful and therefore illegal drug. Such a stand is possible if lawmakers, law enforcement agencies, and educational institutions make a concerted effort not only to learn the dangers of marijuana, but to educate offenders concerning these harms. At the present time, no such effort is being made commensurate with the magnitude of the problem.

In California, for example, the new liberalized law provides that when an offender has been apprehended three or more times for simple possession of marijuana within a two-year period, rather than pay his fine, he may be diverted into an appropriate community program for "education, treatment, or rehabilitation." Since it is easy to avoid apprehension, it is unlikely that many marijuana users in California will ever have to enter a drug education program. It is unlikely that any great percentage of those who use marijuana will ever receive even one citation, let alone be apprehended three times in two years.

A program of education about marijuana founded on the evidence of the drug's long-term effects and the immediate danger of its use in terms of perception and motor coordination (most specifically, the impairment of driving ability) would help enormously. The education program should be offered to both users and nonusers, for I have found that presenting people with real evidence and facts, not hearsay, about marijuana persuades them not to start using marijuana or to stop using it.

One argument given for the legalization of marijuana is that its use would then decrease. Laws against marijuana use are compared with the prohibition against alcohol in the 1920s. To the contrary, facts show that when drugs are readily available, their use increases. In the United States, alcohol consumption declined during Prohibition and rose after repeal of the Eighteenth Amendment (Figure 3); use of heroin and cannabis increased greatly in the armed forces in Germany and Vietnam, where supplies were plentiful and cheap. Amphetamines were widely used by soldiers during World War II to counteract drowsiness and fatigue. After the war, surpluses appeared on the market. In several countries where the drug was then readily available, civilian use of amphetamines escalated. In Japan, a country that had never before had a serious drug problem, amphetamine use rose when army surplus supplies appeared on the black market and when prescriptions were given liberally. By 1954, 500,000 to 600,000 young Japanese were using amphetamines, and half of these had progressed to intravenous injection. Through government control and strict law en-

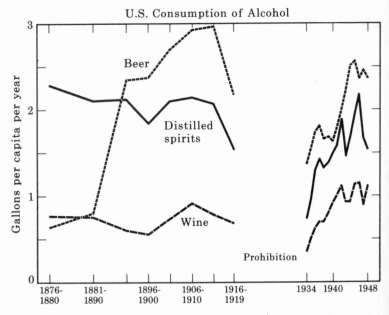

Figure 3. Alcohol consumption in the United States, 1876–1948. Public opinion and education against the use of alcohol are reflected in the decline in consumption during the years immediately preceding ratification of the Eighteenth Amendment in 1919. Following repeal of the amendment in 1933, alcohol consumption rose over a ten-year period. (Data from Patrick, 1952)

forcement, amphetamine abuse was essentially eliminated in Japan by 1968. Even in 1973, when drug abuse was high on college campuses in the United States and many other parts of the world, I observed no evidence of drug abuse among the students on the campuses of Kyoto and Tokyo universities. Physicians at the University Student Health Services in Kyoto confirmed this observation. Although marijuana and some other drugs are reportedly now being used in Japan, law enforcement has contained them (with the exception of solvent sniffing, discussed in Chapter 5).

In Sweden, on an experimental basis, opiates and amphetamines were legally prescribed from 1965 to 1967 to about 200 addicts. Records show that these people received health insurance and social welfare allowances on a larger scale and for longer periods than before. They were unemployed more than previously and had a higher crime rate. During the 1960s the drug policy in general in Sweden was liberal: drugs were overprescribed and easy to obtain. Drug abuse accelerated. It is reported that, with a return to restrictive policies in 1967, the acceleration was checked; when intensified restrictions were introduced in 1969, the rate of abuse fell.

In 1973, Oregon became the first state to change its marijuana laws. At the time the change was made, the National Drug Abuse Council commissioned a market research firm in Portland, Bardsley & Haslacher, Inc., to study patterns of marijuana use for two years. The council concluded from the surveys that marijuana use and attitudes toward it had remained much the same as before. The 1974 survey figures show, however, that out of 802 persons interviewed, 69 were using marijuana; of these 4 had begun using it after the laws were changed. This is an increase of 6 percent. The 1975 survey shows that out of 802 persons interviewed, 65 were using marijuana; of these 9 had begun using it after the laws were changed. This is an increase of 16 percent for the twenty-four-month period following the enactment of the new laws. The numbers of marijuana users interviewed in these surveys are too small to determine accurately the increase in the number of users. However, the numbers are sufficient to establish by statistical inference that the increase in new users could be as high as 18 percent per year (95 percent confidence limit) for the period under study. The survey included only subjects who were eighteen or over. However, in determining the increase in drug use, it must be remembered that people under eighteen are more susceptible to drug use. In 1974, in a small-scale survey of my own of students of several Oregon college campuses, I found that marijuana use among undergraduates had increased by 12.3 percent during the year following revision of Oregon's marijuana laws.

Marijuana use in Oregon has definitely increased since the new laws were put into effect. The only questions remaining are the magnitude of the increase and whether the trend is different from what it would have been if the law had not been changed. Several other states have recently reduced their penalties for possession of marijuana, and more extensive studies will probably be done. Reliable results will, however, take years to obtain.

Perhaps more definitive than the statistics are the attitudes, especially of students I interviewed in Oregon, concerning the status of marijuana. All those I interviewed believed that marijuana had been "legalized" in Oregon. They were aware of the distinction between decriminalization and legalization, but they felt the drug had been legalized for practical purposes and it was just a question of time until the legal barriers would be fully removed. No one knew, for example, of a single person who had been fined under the new law.

As marijuana use is allowed to spread, other problems that have not yet been generally recognized will be magnified. Of major importance to everyone is the effect of increased marijuana use on the automobile accident rate. The concern of the Canadian government about this problem was an important factor in its decision to oppose decriminalization. Some interesting tests have shown that marijuana definitely impairs driving ability (Davis, 1970; Klein *et al.*, 1971). Students who smoked less than twice a week reported they had some difficulty driving and tried not to drive when they had been smoking. Students who smoked more than twice a week and who were habitual users tended to play down any difficulty they had in driving. Either they wanted to defend their use of marijuana or they were less aware that their driving ability had been impaired.

One of the most dramatic tests for impaired driving ability involved the monitoring by tape recorder of a driver who had smoked two and a half joints. He was accompanied by a control. The following are excerpts from the tape:

I now feel my head vibrating in between two and three different people. I forgot to look one way when I rounded that corner. I went into third gear very, very poorly, possibly the worst I've done in my entire life. I am coming to a stop sign, and for some reason I feel maybe I won't be able to stop. It's difficult to force my foot down to the floor on the brake. It seems as though both my feet are riding on cushions, the cushions between my feet and the brake pedal. . . .

I feel as though I'm riding high in my seat. The lane seems quite wide enough but the car cannot go fast enough, and it appears miles to the next stop. I seem to have different . . . I seem to sway back and forth across the road. . . .

I'm very frightened of cars passing me. . . . I cannot handle this curve much longer, 'cause I feel like I'm going around the edge of a teacup, and I hate going around the edge of a teacup in a car. It's like I'm going to roll right off, it's like I'm way up on top of the world. I'm really frightened up here – it's so very high. Oh, it's like going straight down [road was actually flat]. . . . I've got to say something – I cannot possibly drive now, no matter what anyone does to me because I am driving on my head. You know, driving is not good when you are upside down, folks, and us – I have to get off the road – my God, what was happening. [Davis, 1970]

The driver pulled off the road. By chance, a highway patrolman came along to see why they had stopped. The driver and control changed places, explaining that they had driven some distance and the driver was tired. The policeman left; he had not detected that the driver was high on marijuana.

The second tape of the study was just as convincing. In this experiment, three youths, all high on marijuana, were in the car. They had some of the same problems as the driver in the first experiment. In addition, while they were driving along the highway, one of the occupants opened his door and tried to get out. The driver thought it was a great joke and kept on going. He had no sense of danger.

Rushes of distracting thought have been reported by automobile drivers under the influence of marijuana. In one study (Klein *et al.*, 1971) a driver testified: "Your mind wanders off to something else." Another driver said: "I think it is too easy to forget that you are driving a car. It is easy to become distracted by music or lights."

Although drunk driving is still the primary cause of traffic accidents, marijuana use is beginning to be identified as a significant factor. In one study, fourteen persons admitted to the emergency room of Denver General Hospital who had been in single-car accidents and charged with operating a motor vehicle under the influence of drugs were given laboratory tests to verify drug use. In six persons, test results were positive for alcohol alone; in five, for marijuana alone; in one, for marijuana and opiates; and in two, for opiates alone (Kier, 1975).

Another study examined drivers "most responsible" for fatal traffic accidents. Using 267 traffic deaths in which drug use could be verified as a cause, the researcher found that 9 percent of the accidents could be directly attributed to marijuana; 18 percent were caused by drivers who had used a combination of alcohol and marijuana; another 4 percent were caused by drivers who had used a combination of alcohol, marijuana, and street pharmaceutical drugs; and 57 percent involved alcohol alone (Sterling-Smith, 1975). Of special significance is the fact that 45 percent of all drivers "most responsible" for fatalities were smokers of marijuana and 19 percent more had experimented with the drug. The effects of marijuana use on this 45 percent undoubtedly added to effects of other drugs taken. Thus, marijuana must have contributed to more accidents than the 9 percent attributed to it.

Exactly what part marijuana plays in accidents due to multiple drug use is difficult to establish; however, one study demonstrated that two drinks of alcohol plus a moderate dose of marijuana can cause heavy intoxication. A study sponsored by the Insurance Bureau of Canada (Burford *et al.*, 1975; Smiley *et al.*, 1975) showed that alcohol at a blood level of 0.06 percent (less than the legal impairment level in Canada, which is 0.08 percent) plus a moderate dose of marijuana increased impairment so that subjects drove (on simulated driving machines) as if their blood level of alcohol was more than 0.1 percent.

What must now be examined in detail is the effect of *chronic* marijuana use on driving ability. Since persistent effects of the drug are known to include impaired judgment, lower attention span, poor perceptions of time, distance, and speed, and defective motor coordination, it seems likely that even between highs a chronic marijuana user's driving ability is impaired. This can be better tested when practical methods for determining the THC content in the body become available.

Deaths due to accidents have shown increases that correspond to the increasing use of drugs in the United States. For many years, there was a downward trend in accidental deaths; but in the mid-1960s, a reversal occurred abruptly among those fifteen to thirty-five years old. The accidental death rate in this age group increased approximately 30 percent between 1961 and 1971, and the automobile accidental death rate increased over 30 percent in the same time period. The increase in these ten years first appeared in college-aged persons; in later years, it spread to younger and older age groups, corresponding precisely with the ages affected by the drug movement in the United States (see Appendix 11).

An increase in the accident rate among the marijuana users is also beginning to show up in the records of emergency treatment centers. According to the Drug Enforcement Administration of the U.S. Department of Justice: "Data from 790 hospital emergency rooms around the country reveal a 20 percent rise in emergency-room episodes involving marijuana from the first quarter of 1974 to the fourth quarter. In about 40 percent of these episodes, the only drug involved was marijuana; 60 percent of the cases involved marijuana and other substances" (Jenson, in U.S. Senate Hearings, 1975).

It is especially important to look more deeply into the long-range implications of legalizing marijuana. To do this, we can examine countries where marijuana has been used for centuries. Most of these countries now have severe laws against the use of marijuana. South Africa, Brazil, Turkey, and Greece, where the use of cannabis was commonplace, supported the Egyptian proposal at the Second Opium Conference (1924) to list cannabis as a dangerous drug. The United Nations Single Convention (1961) stated that marijuana was a harmful drug and included cannabis among the concerns for the control of narcotic and stupefying drugs. The United States is a party to the agreement to "limit exclusively to medical and scientific purposes, the production, manufacture, export, import, distribution of, trade in, use and possession of drugs" covered by the convention. The Geneva Conference of the International Narcotics Control Commission (1975) confirmed the stand taken originally in 1961.

It is especially important to consider the international implications if the United States takes a permissive stand on marijuana. Many people in our Justice Department feel that if our marijuana laws are relaxed too far, our positions on harder narcotic drugs will be in jeopardy in terms of our agreements with other countries.

It is interesting to note, as has one Swedish authority, that "demand for legalizing cannabis has been strongest in those countries which have had the shortest experience and the weakest forms of the drug" (Bejerot, in U.S. Senate Hearings, 1974). In all the twenty-one countries my wife and I visited during a study of drug abuse problems, and particularly in the countries where cannabis use is endemic, people were dismayed to hear of the attempts in the United States to legalize marijuana. They felt that legalization would allow drug use to spread through the entire population. In countries where cannabis has long been used, it is considered a scourge, a stupefying drug especially harmful to youth; and it is felt to be a factor in keeping the poor impoverished. "In the countries of endemic cannabis intoxication the widespread use of the drug by the working class is associated with inefficiency and social stagnation" (Nahas, 1973). These countries try to keep cannabis use from spreading from the subpopulation of chronic users to the general population.

Although the obvious problems are recognizable in a nation of cannabis-smokers, research needs to be done on the hidden dangers. Some attribute the poor health of the cannabis-using populations solely to inadequate nutrition and health care and ignore the possible effects of cannabis itself. Unfortunately, adequate vital statistics are lacking for such populations. The available statistics indicate, however, that persons in the lower socioeconomic groups in countries where cannabis use is heavy show early degenerative changes and are likely to produce a higher-than-usual proportion of defective offspring. Fortunately, females are not the main users of cannabis in these populations. The children are thus spared the risk of exposure to THC before birth. However, the incidence of birth defects in these populations is high, and in view of the recent findings on chromosome and gene damage, it is not unlikely that cannabis is a cause. It must be remembered, too, when considering the genetic effects of marijuana on a population, that damaged genes usually cause no specific, observable defect, but rather a general decline in physical and mental vigor, which is passed on to offspring.

As a nation we should not consider ourselves immune to the harmful effects of marijuana. Speaking on this point, Zeidenberg stated (in U.S. Senate Hearings, 1974) that "to regard ourselves as immune to this syndrome is not only potentially destructive to our society but an affront to our foreign neighbors who have more pragmatic experience with this problem and with whom we have existing treaties to outlaw this drug." Not only do we have an obligation to other countries and this generation of young people, we must also consider how our laws and attitudes will affect future generations. Louria has put it well:

Currently, we have three major legal drugs of pleasure, caffeine, nicotine, and alcohol. Caffeine is relatively safe; nicotine is said to cost us between 60,000 and 300,000 deaths and $19 billion in economic loss each year; alcohol costs us at least 40,000 and probably nearer 100,000 lives yearly, and at least $15 billion in economic loss per year. The question is, Do we wish to add a fourth intoxicant, marijuana, to our other three? If we do legalize marijuana, we will impose this fourth intoxicant on our children, grandchildren, and great-grandchildren, for once a new intoxicant is legitimatized and accepted by the public, it cannot subsequently be arbitrarily proscribed. This is what we learned from Prohibition. [Louria, in U.S. Senate Hearings, 1974]

The pressure for the legalization of marijuana so soon after we have begun to understand its chemistry, pharmacology, and toxicology is strong. Although some states have claimed that they are relaxing their marijuana laws for a trial period, Zeidenberg, like Louria, considered legalization an irreversible legislative step:

I use the term "irreversible" deliberately, because I wish to emphasize that legalization of use of an agent in society creates a situation in which the agent becomes embedded in the social structure and is virtually impossible to extirpate. One need only look at the situation in regard to alcohol and cigarettes to realize this obvious fact. . . . There is no question in my mind that legalization of marijuana will lead to a large population of chronic heavy marijuana users, numbering in the millions, just as prevails with alcohol and tobacco. Both of these latter agents exact a terrifying toll in human life, suffering and expense in this country annually. I think it is probable that heavy marijuana use in our country would create a third at-risk population overlapping only in part with the two previous groups and further add to mortality, morbidity and public cost. [Zeidenberg, in U.S. Senate Hearings, 1974]

The government of Canada has resisted efforts in that country to legalize marijuana. The minister of national health and welfare, Marc La Londe, wrote:

The government of Canada is not prepared to give legal sanction to the use of cannabis. Cannabis use carries with it social, psychological and physical hazards which the government is not prepared to see become more widespread and more serious. Nor, as far as I can determine from the overwhelming majority of letters sent to my office, do the people of Canada want to see cannabis legalized. . . . The government is concerned about marijuana's potential for harm in the safe operation of motor vehicles and machinery, in relation to brain and chromosome damage, and on the maturation process, and that is why Bill S-19 [introducing modification of the marijuana laws] does not propose the legalization or decriminalization of cannabis. [*Toronto Star*, 1975]

The main objection to our old marijuana laws is that, when enforced, they give marijuana users criminal records. The problem for lawmakers, then, is how to structure more humane and enforceable laws that at the same time effectively discourage use of marijuana. This is a difficult task and one that carries tremendous responsibilities. Even the decriminalization of marijuana raises some difficult questions both in drafting the law and in its enforcement. What about the use of these drugs by minors? What about hashish and the concentrated product, cannabis oil? Is synthetic THC legal, too? Should LSD, psilocybin, and mescaline also be decriminalized, since they are comparable in potency to THC? When considering marijuana use, we must also realize that Americans are consuming not only greater quantities of marijuana but stronger varieties of cannabis preparations. As DuPont has testified (in U.S. Senate Hearings, 1975): "There appears to be a large and growing minority who use the drug more frequently, at higher potency, and at a younger age. These trends disturb even the most optimistic observers of the contemporary marijuana scene in this country." We are no longer talking about the mild marijuana cited by the La Guardia Report or even that used at the time of the Shafer Commission study, but about much more potent varieties. As shown earlier, 85 percent of the marijuana smokers in my spring 1976 sample of college males had smoked hashish one or more times. In my first sampling in 1968, none had. How will the law handle the wide range in the strength of the varieties of cannabis and its different preparations? What is the legal "intoxicating" dose of THC? Should any legislation be attempted without a practical means for objectively determining the degree of exposure?

Considering the possibility of flashbacks in the marijuana user and the effects present between highs, will those responsible for the lives of others, such as airplane pilots and surgeons, be allowed to use marijuana? If so, how much? How will the amount be measured? Will the people for whom they are responsible have the right to be informed of this use of marijuana? Also to be considered are the variation in effects among individuals and the compound effects from even small doses of marijuana used in combination with alcohol, stimulant drugs, or some medications.

In amending our marijuana laws to make them more humane and constructive, we must not lose sight of the real dangers and the stand which the government must take against them. Enough has been proved already in animal studies alone to warrant caution. In fact, on the basis of such damaging evidence, even from animal studies alone, any other new substance being considered for human use would be banned immediately.

Real research on marijuana has just begun. Only a few of the ingredients in marijuana have been tested for their biological effects. Of the fifty cannabinoids identified, only Δ-9-THC has been tested extensively in its purified state. Even for THC, we probably know only a few of its effects in cells; we are far from understanding *how* it affects cellular and subcellular functions. Undoubtedly, additional research will further establish that other chemical constituents in marijuana also affect biological systems. Such research takes time. Nearly a century of scientific work has gone into the study of the effects of aspirin and of opiates on the nervous system, and we still cannot completely explain how they act on cellular functions.

Research is being done to discover medical uses for marijuana. I believe, however, that its use as a medicine will be limited. Other drugs now being prescribed as anticonvulsants, analgesics, and tranquilizers, and as treatments for glaucoma and asthma, are effective and have fewer detrimental side effects than marijuana. Even if a medical use is discovered, marijuana will not be any safer to use as a sensual drug.

At the beginning of the movement in the United States (in the 1960s) to legalize marijuana, advocates used to say marijuana was a harmless drug; I saw many young people start smoking it on this assumption. As more evidence was presented to the contrary, the advocates changed their arguments. "Marijuana," they said, "is no more harmful than alcohol, which is legal." They continued: "Everyone has the right to do what he pleases with regard to personal drug use." Now that evidence indicates the possibility of fetal damage from marijuana use, the advocates say that no drug is completely harmless and that, like any drug, marijuana should be used with caution by pregnant women. The advocates still deny that marijuana has been proved to alter chromosomes, damage the lungs or the brain, affect DNA or RNA, or suppress the immune system. However, they now say that such facts are "controversial." Nevertheless, advocates of liberalization of the marijuana laws say they cannot wait for more research because the laws are "making criminals out of our children." It is clear that advocates have had to change their arguments with the appearance of each new piece of evidence against marijuana.

Even when advocates of decriminalization admit that marijuana may be harmful, they do not propound these warnings to the public. For example, Stroup, director of the National Organization for the Reform of the Marijuana Laws (as reported by DuPont, in U.S. Senate Hearings, 1975), has said that "there are enough unanswered medical questions to warn against [marijuana] use." However, this statement has had little publicity, and the organization continues actively campaigning for the elimination of the legal restrictions against the use of marijuana.

It is the responsibility of the lawmakers to inform themselves about the dangers of marijuana use and to take a public stand. Indeed, those lawmakers who advocate decriminalization of marijuana have a particular responsibility to implement the recommendation of the Shafer Commission that "society should continue actively to discourage people from using marijuana."

One lawmaker, defending his vote for the decriminalization of marijuana in California, was quoted as saying that the marijuana laws were inconsistent and failed to "effectively deter usage of marijuana." Furthermore, he stated that "regardless of how stringent the laws are, if parents fail to teach that excessive use of drugs has adverse effects upon health, no law or penalty will be able to force good health upon these children." His statements are true enough, but he sidestepped the issue and overlooked both the important role law could play in controlling drug abuse and his own responsibility to legislate such laws.

The law is, in fact, a deterrent. In a sample of 2,000 twenty-three-year-old males, former marijuana users most often cited concern about being arrested as their main reason for discontinuing drug use. Among those who never smoked marijuana, this concern was most often third on the list of reasons for not starting (DuPont, in U.S. Senate Hearings, 1975).

A weakening of the marijuana laws means to many people that authorities consider the drug safe. In my opinion, any new marijuana law should contain the information that marijuana is a harmful drug and should not be used. More importantly, the law should make provision for the dissemination of this information. If marijuana use is to be stopped, we need both laws and education. We must legislate, not for overly harsh punishment or for permissive neglect, but for effective education.

The problem, then, seems to be one of informing the public of the real facts. As Kolansky and Moore (1975) stated: "To date, most of the public remains uninformed about medical findings that clearly indicate substantial health hazards as a result of marijuana smoking. A systematic campaign to disseminate medical information is long overdue, particularly by governmental agencies and the news media."

In the past decade, many studies and government reports on marijuana use have been biased by the political movement to legalize the drug. For example, studies were made of short-term effects, experiments were conducted using weak marijuana, subjects were preselected for their relative good health, and the results of inappropriate tests have been cited as evidence that marijuana use is harmless. Reports have sometimes been ambiguous and have obscured the facts. As a result, the public has been confused. For example, the following statement was treated merely as a footnote in the annual report to the president by the Domestic Council Drug Abuse Task Force (1975): "Recent research indicates that marijuana is far from harmless, and . . . chronic use can produce adverse psychological and physiological effects. Therefore, its use should be strongly discouraged as a matter of national policy." However, in the main text of this report, marijuana was described as having the least serious consequences of all the sensual drugs. It was also the only sensual drug rated low in all three of the following: (1) likelihood that a user will become physically or psychologically dependent, (2) severity of adverse consequences to the individual, (3) severity of adverse consequences to society. Unless the reader found the footnote (in fine print), he would assume that the task force considered marijuana to be a harmless drug. As another example, the staff of the Shafer Commission have been criticized for the manner in which they placed words and paragraphs together in writing the commission's report on marijuana – either unintentionally or as "a calculated effort to distract attention from the report's strong cautionary language" (Cowan, in U.S. Senate Hearings, 1974).

Each year I receive hundreds of requests for information about the dangers of marijuana use from the people most responsible for educating the youth of this country: teachers, religious leaders, military personnel, doctors, and nurses. By far the largest number of letters comes from concerned parents. I was contacted recently by the father of a teenage boy who, with three of his friends, had been caught smoking marijuana. The police, rather than arresting the boys, had given them warning citations and assigned them to write papers on marijuana. The boys checked out the books available on marijuana at the local library. These contained information on how to identify marijuana, where it is grown, the various grades and forms of marijuana, how they are used, who uses them, and the social implications of use; but nothing definitive on the harmful effects of marijuana use.

The evening after his son had been cited, the father saw me on a television debate and decided to contact me. He told me that his older daughters, now out of college and not marijuana users, had been arguing for marijuana for years, insisting that the drug had no proved harmful effects, that it was no more harmful than alcohol, and that the worst effect was from antiquated laws that made criminals out of young people. The father had no evidence to prove them wrong and was beginning to think he was out of date and that, perhaps, marijuana was a harmless drug.

For several weeks before the boy was apprehended, his mother and father had been worried because he was losing interest in his studies and his usual activities and was becoming antagonistic at home. The father said they had attributed his problems to "growing up." That the boy might be using marijuana had flashed through the father's mind, but the idea had been dismissed, since the family was close and there was no evidence of marijuana use.

The father was not satisfied with the material available at the library and asked me for source material. He was particularly impressed with the collection of the scientific evidence on the effects of marijuana presented at the U.S. Senate hearings in 1974 (see Appendix 8). He found it unbelievable that such extensive, sound information had not been given wide public exposure. Popular articles reviewing reports on the harmful effects of marijuana available in various scientific magazines (Fisher, 1975; Maugh, 1975) were also used. (A practical information booklet has recently been written on the subject [Russell, 1975].) His son pored over the material and wrote his paper. In the descriptions of the effects of marijuana, the boy recognized his own friends. He also saw that his family's observations of his behavioral changes had been true. He decided to stop smoking marijuana.

Fortunately, this father had a good relationship with his son; he did not ignore or try to justify his son's marijuana use with such commonly heard excuses as "all the kids are doing it." He made an effort to find the facts. He took a definite stand against marijuana use, and just as importantly, worked with his son to find a solution.

I give this example not only to show a typical case, but to show that parents can be effective in stopping drug use. In fact, they are one of the most important influences in forming their children's attitudes. DuPont has said that the breakup of the traditional, close-knit American family has contributed significantly to the rise in teenage drug abuse. Children are also influenced by their parents' drug use. A study of 8,000 New York high school students (Kandel, 1973) disclosed that the adolescents most likely to use marijuana were those whose best friends were users and whose parents used psychoactive drugs – including tranquilizers, sedatives, and diet and pep pills.

Teachers are important influences also. In my university class on drug abuse, students who have stopped using marijuana long enough to notice the difference often bring their friends to my class or office for a conference in an attempt to get the friends to abandon marijuana use also.

The goal of drug laws is not to stigmatize offenders. The goal is rather to provide education so that the vast majority will understand the hazards and avoid drug abuse. The legal remedies needed in the United States are those that will educate against use and present a steady deterrent against the drug epidemic.

Appendixes

Effect of drugs on mental state

The effects of the psychoactive substances listed in Table 11 are determined by concentration of the substance on the brain cell membrane. These substances are not highly specific for the membrane, but when taken in sufficient quantities they accumulate on the membrane. THC

Table 11. *Relation of mental state and body content of psychoactive substances that accumulate on cell surface and interfere with cell membrane function*[a]

| Substance | Amount (grams) producing | | | |
	Normal state	Mild intoxi- cation	Heavy intoxi- cation	Uncon- sciousness
Low fat/water solubility ratio				
Nitrogen (N_2 dissolved in body tissue)				
Sea level	1.7			
Deep sea				
10 atm		17		
28 atm			50	
100 atm				170
Nitrous oxide	0	1–2	4–20	70
Ethylene	0	0.5	1	2
Cyclopropane	0	0.4	1	2
Ethyl alcohol	Trace	50	100	250
Ethyl ether	0	1	4	8
Very high fat/water solubility ratio				
THC (cannabis)	0	0.005	0.2	1

[a] Estimates for a 70-kilogram man.
Source: Adapted from Goodman and Gilman (1975); Jones (1950).

(the active principle in marijuana) produces similar effects, but with one one-thousandth the intake. This is because THC becomes highly concentrated in fat and in the lipid structures of the cell membrane.

The psychoactive substances listed in Table 12 have low fat/water solubility ratios; their principal effect is on the brain cell enzymes that regulate neuron activation.

Table 12. *Relation of mental state and body content of psychoactive substances that specifically affect brain cell enzymes*[a]

Substance	Amount (grams) producing			
	Normal state	Mild intoxi- cation	Heavy intoxi- cation	Uncon- sciousness
Morphine[c]	0	0.003	0.01	0.04
Heroin[c]	0	0.001	0.004	0.01
Barbiturates	0	0.03	0.10	0.5–1.0
Cocaine	0	0.03	0.1[b]	0.5[b]
Amphetamine sulfate	0	0.02–0.04	0.04–0.1[b]	
Diazepam (Valium)	0	0.005		
Ephedrine	0	0.05	0.1[b]	
Adrenaline[c]	0.00001	0.0001	0.0005[b]	
Atropine	0	0.002	0.005	0.01
LSD-25	0	0.00002	0.0002	

[a] Estimates for a normal 70-kilogram man.
[b] This amount is associated with risk of vascular occlusion or hemorrhage.
[c] Injected
Source: Adapted from Goodman and Gilman (1975).

Fate of marijuana in the body

THC: fat solubility and resistance to metabolism

Some of the effects of marijuana on cells and tissues are related to the physical molecular properties of the cannabinoids. A distinctive property of the cannabinoids is their high solubility in fat and low solubility in water. The principal active cannabinoid of marijuana, THC (tetrahydrocannabinol), is 6,000 times more soluble in fat than in water; other cannabinoids, including most of the partially degraded products of THC formed in the body, show a similar characteristic (Gill *et al.*, 1972, 1973). THC associates with fats in the body. The effects of anesthetic drugs are roughly proportional to fat/water solubility ratios, but the maximum ratios of these are usually only a few hundred to one.

The effect of marijuana on the body is also determined by the drug's chemical molecular properties: THC is not completely metabolized. Cannabinoid molecules, unlike most organic substances, are not fully oxidized into carbon dioxide and water. They remain cannabinoid residues with properties similar to those of THC. With each fresh exposure to THC, it is carried in the blood in a form that is initially excreted by the kidneys, but this phase of removal is over by the time one-third, or less, of the THC has collected in the urine. From this stage, the THC and residues are bound tightly to fat and are not excreted by the urine but are slowly excreted by the bile.

Bile is a watery fluid, secreted by the liver, that flows into the intestine. It contains bile salts and other materials. The biliary system plays an important part in the transport, digestion, and excretion of fat-soluble substances. The bile salts combine with these fat-soluble substances so that they become water-soluble or emulsified and dispersed in water; these complexes are the means both for eliminating toxic fat-soluble

301

substances and for absorbing fats in digestion of food. Bile transports fat-complexed residues needing excretion from the blood and the liver to the intestinal cavity. There the bile salts separate from the fat wastes carried from the body and then combine with the fats released by digestive enzymes, which are absorbed with the bile salts into the body. Recirculation of bile salts is the body's fat-excretion and fat-absorption system. Bile salt recirculation among the blood, the liver, and the intestine is the means, for example, of eliminating excess quantities of cholesterol from the body. It is also the way cannabinoids are excreted.

The original discovery that the active ingredient of hemp is fat-soluble should be credited to some unknown Indian who long ago found that the psychic ingredient in hemp could be extracted by butter and to the first chemist, also unknown, who found it could be extracted by petrol-ether. The significance of the fat solubility of THC was discovered recently by Gill and Jones working in Paton's laboratory. Their quantitation of the fat/water solubility ratio established the unusually high value for THC. Paton and his colleagues have used the unusually high fat uptake of THC and other cannabinoids as a basis for predicting and understanding the adverse effects on cells – especially cells of brain tissue. Motivated by Paton's early ideas about the uptake of THC by the brain, Campbell *et al.* (1971) found evidence of cerebral atrophy in heavy users of marijuana. There can be no doubt that fat solubility and incomplete metabolic degradation account for the long retention of cannabinoids in the body and their accumulation in lipid structures of cell membranes.

The fat/water solubility ratio of THC is close to that of gasoline and jet fuel. But the only similarity between THC and these substances is that, when taken into the body, they migrate to the fat. The average person is exposed to much more kerosene vapor at airports and to more gasoline vapor at automobile service stations than the marijuana smoker is exposed to THC. The petroleum products have no apparent psychic effect when 5 milligrams is absorbed into the body or when 10 micrograms is taken into the brain, where the resultant concentration is 10 parts per billion. This, however, is the average THC intake of the marijuana smoker. Hence, though fat solubility is one of the keys to the action and long-term retention of THC, other properties determine its psychoactive characteristics. This is further emphasized by the fact that another cannabinoid, cannabidiol, is not appreciably psychoactive despite its high fat/water solubility ratio (Paton *et al.*, 1972). The psychic action of THC (and its more psychoactive metabolite, 11-hydroxy-THC) appears related to specific effects on the lipid phases of cell structures.

THC: distribution and retention

The fate of THC in the body has been discovered by means of studies of laboratory animals and humans. THC labeled with a radioactive isotope (either tritium or carbon 14) has been administered and traced in the body. Distribution, retention, transformation to other chemical forms (metabolites), and excretion have been determined in this way.

Retention of labeled THC in humans was found to be 40 percent at 3 days; 30 percent at 1 week (Lemberger *et al.*, 1971,1972), and by extrapolation, 10 percent at 48 days, and 1 percent at 4.6 months. Similarly high retention was found in laboratory rodents (McIsaac *et al.*, 1971; Klausner & Dingell, 1971; Harbison & Mantilla-Plata, 1972; Kreuz & Axelrod, 1973). Behavior is comparable in mice, rats, and humans, except that small animals are more active per unit of size, and the time of retention is correspondingly reduced. There are also minor species differences in the patterns of partial breakdown of THC prior to excretion as cannabinol residues.

In the typical animal study, labeled THC was administered in measured amounts sufficient to produce acute intoxication (Harbison & Mantilla-Plata, 1972). During the initial period following intraperitoneal injection of THC, the concentration of THC was highest in the blood and viscera, where the maximum levels were found within an hour. The levels then began to fall at a rate of 2 to 3 percent per minute, decreasing by half every thirty minutes or so. When the levels decreased to about 25 percent of peak concentration, they began to decline much more slowly (approximately by half in the next thirty hours rather than in thirty minutes). The period of high concentration in the blood and viscera, as well as the brain, corresponds to the period of acute intoxication, lasting two to six hours in both laboratory animals and humans. When THC is injected directly into the blood, peak concentrations occur at once (Klausner & Dingell, 1971; Lemberger *et al.*, 1972). The slower rise from smoking marijuana, a lag of at least fifteen minutes, has to do with the absorption of THC from carbon particles that carry it into the lungs. When marijuana is absorbed through the gut rather than smoked or injected, THC appearing in the blood is more extensively metabolized to the more psychoactive 11-hydroxy-THC (Lemberger *et al.*, 1972). Persons who have eaten marijuana report that the high starts later and lasts somewhat longer than when they smoked the same amount.

The level of THC in the blood decreases after reaching its peak partly because of uptake by fatty tissue and partly because a small fraction of the

THC is excreted in the urine during the first few days (Lemberger *et al.*, 1970, 1971, 1972). This phenomenon suggests that at first not all the THC enters the blood-fat transport system. Part of it is excreted before it can dissolve in THC-retaining lipids. The major factor, however, in the reduction of blood levels of THC is the transfer of the drug from the blood into tissue and cell fat. Because of the varying fat content of the different tissues of the body, the ratio of THC (or its metabolites) absorbed by adipose tissue (50 percent fat) to that absorbed by lean tissue (1 percent fat) is actually only about 50:1, the ratio of fat content. This is far from the oil/water solubility ratio of 6000:1, but it is still a large ratio. In the average man, whose body is 17 percent fat, the uptake of THC by fatty tissue is 90 percent. It must be kept in mind, however, that a large part of the remaining 10 percent of THC is in the fat that constitutes part of all cells, especially the cell membranes. Within fat structures of cell membranes, THC concentrates 6,000 times more than in the adjacent water phase. Paton (1975) has reviewed the evidence showing that the THC concentrates in membranes of brain cells and red blood cells 600 and 380 times greater, respectively, than in the blood plasma. If the blood plasma did not contain fat bound to proteins and if the portions of the membrane that are fat could have been measured, the ratios should have been 10 to 16 times higher or 6000:1.

In the lean body, fat is mostly bound to protein, forming compounds called *lipoproteins*. Excess fat does occur unbound in the form of oil droplets ballooning out each fat cell. Lipoproteins are responsible for the transport of fat in the blood and other body fluids. The outer membrane of each cell must have contact with both the fat and the water phases of body parts, and this is provided by lipoproteins in the cell membrane. In simple terms, the protein component contributes to the membrane's permeability to water-soluble substances, and the lipid component contributes to its permeability to fat-soluble substances. THC alters the lipid properties of the cell membrane.

The transport of fat by lipoproteins is subject to variation from person to person because of differences in quantities of the various lipoproteins of blood. These differences may account for differences in individual patterns of distribution and retention of THC and perhaps for differences in sensitivity to marijuana. The movement of labeled THC into and out of the blood is much faster than the turnover or replacement of lipoproteins; thus, it appears that THC, like other substances transported by lipoproteins, moves into and out of the lipoproteins depending on the rate of its transfer from the blood lipoproteins into tissue.

The uptake of THC by fat occurs at a rate determined by the quantity of blood flowing through the fatty tissue per unit of time. The THC evidently moves freely from the lipoproteins of the blood into the cell fat (including the large droplets of fat in fat storage cells) until the concentrations of THC in the two systems are proportional to their fat content. As the THC concentration in the blood is reduced by the slow removal of THC from the blood by bile, the fat cells disgorge some of their THC content back into the blood. The slow blood flow through fatty tissue, the large capacity of fat for THC, and the slow elimination via the bile into the feces combine to cause the THC to be retained in the body for long periods. With repeated exposures, THC accumulates not only in adipose tissue but in the membranes of all body cells as well.

THC: effects on cell membranes

Although the peak concentration of THC in the blood and in the brain, with the accompanying psychic symptoms, is of short duration and is followed by a rapid decline, the concentration does not become negligible for a very long time. Measuring the concentration of THC in the brain as a whole yields a value lower than in most other tissues; but this fact is misleading, and it must be remembered, as mentioned above, that the concentrations in the cell membranes (where critical events of nervous activity take place) will be far higher. The high concentration of THC in the brain cell membranes probably accounts for the immediate intoxication and for the long-term changes in brain function, for it is the brain cell membrane that provides intercellular contacts.

The presence of THC in the lipid structures of cell membranes causes some dislocation in these structures. Cannabidiol and cannabinol, which are also absorbed after smoking marijuana, affect the membranes and function of liver cells (Paton *et al.*, 1972; Paton & Pertwee, 1973*b*). Some effects of THC on brain and liver cell membranes are similar to those of alcohol and anesthetics (Paton *et al.*, 1972). There is, however, an important difference between the effects of alcohol and of THC: the effect of THC in altering cell membrane structure occurs with *small* exposures to THC, and there is a cutoff level above which the effect does not increase. The interpretation of this cutoff is that the strong absorption of THC by the lipids of the cell membrane is quenched when the sites having affinity for THC have been saturated. Although the absorption of THC is essentially a physical attraction, the exceptionally strong binding of THC by lipid makes the absorption resemble a chemical reaction. The presence of THC in cell membranes is responsible for the depression of such processes as protein synthesis, cell division, nucleic acid synthesis, and enzymatic changes (Leuchtenberger, Morishima, Nahas, in U.S. Senate Hearings, 1974).

A consequence of the accumulation of THC in cell membranes is alteration of membrane structure and, by inference, alteration of cell function. The type of change, a *fluidification* of the membrane, has been illustrated by Lawrence and Gill (1975). These investigators prepared artificial *lipid bilayers*, in the form of *liposomes*, obtained by ultrasonic treatment of a mixture of membrane constituents. These were labeled with an electron spin resonance (ESR) marker. On exposure to THC (as with exposure to anesthetics), the change in ESR signal indicated an increase in mobility of the lipid in the membrane.

The observations made by several researchers that THC alters cell membrane structures and functions have been confirmed and greatly extended by Heath. He found that synaptic changes develop in monkeys exposed to marijuana smoke. He observed a significant widening of the synaptic cleft associated with accumulation of radiopaque material and a clumping of the synaptic vesicles – an early sign of neuronal degeneration (see Appendix 9).

THC: accumulation

When radioisotope-labeled THC is given in repeated doses, it accumulates in the tissues and organs, as would be expected from the long retention of THC (Kreuz & Axelrod, 1973). Adipose tissue, of course, shows the most accumulation, but the brain and other body organs also show this effect. In the brain, the increase in THC content is slow but clearly observable over weeks of intake. Particularly interesting is the fact that compounds to which THC is converted also accumulate in the body. When the same amount of THC is administered every other day, the level of THC in the brain after a month appears to be about the same as the transitory peak level immediately after a similar exposure. But there is a very important difference: the retention of THC in the brain is not a transitory event of a few hours' duration, for THC content is already at the level represented by body fat. The accumulated THC is held more tenaciously in the brain tissue. Its elimination then depends on removing the THC residues from the body as a whole – a matter of many months' abstinence for humans.

These findings correspond to the cumulative mental impairment associated with marijuana smoking. The first few exposures have little psychic effect. This is because brain cells must become charged with

THC to the point that an additional but transitory uptake overburdens brain function and produces the high.

Other effects of marijuana

The full story of the effects of marijuana on the body is much more complicated than the story of THC presented here. For example, another cannabinoid of marijuana smoke, cannabidiol, in addition to modifying the lipid structure of the cell membrane differently from THC, impairs liver cell microsomal activity. The suppression of microsomal activity in liver cells causes a general reduction in the ability of the liver to decompose toxic substances (Paton *et al.*, 1972). This is why the use of marijuana accentuates the effect of barbiturates; the liver microsomes are unable to degrade the barbiturate molecules at the usual speed. Cannabidiol does not appear to contribute to the psychic effects of marijuana, but its effect on liver microsomes suggests that marijuana smoking may involve more harm than the studies with purified THC have implied.

Observations on the recovery of blood and vital organs from THC intoxication are deceptive. The rapid loss of THC from the blood and vital organs is merely the result of the transfer of the THC into the fat.

Another consideration, overlooked in most studies, is that THC moves from one body system (or compartment) to another and circulates among compartments in a turnover process at variable rates, some of which are very slow. As THC moves into compartments with slower turnover rates, less of the labeled THC appears in the transfer among compartments. In studies of short duration, the accumulation of very small daily amounts does not become detectable; yet many of the studies have been terminated after only a few days. A different story would become evident if humans were exposed to the labeled THC over a long period of use. It is probable that some of the THC residues with slow turnover rates may account for the clinical symptoms that accumulate slowly and abate only after many months' abstinence.

Some information about opiates

Most commonly abused opiates

Opium. Crude gum from the oriental poppy pod. Opium contains at least twenty known opiate drugs that can be separately extracted. Among them are morphine, codeine, dihydromorphinone (Dilaudid), and papaverine. All affect nerve functions, but vary in primary sites of action. Raw opium has numerous sites of action and can be used medically for relief of severe pain, headaches, and diarrhea. Today, owing to the availability of synthetic replacements and chemically modified opiates, opium is not as essential as it once was in the practice of modern medicine. Before antibiotics, tincture of opium (paregoric) was commonly used to treat diarrhea.

Morphine. The principal natural opiate in opium and the opiate generally used medically for the relief of severe pain.

Codeine. One of the derivatives of opium. Medically it is used to control coughing and to relieve migraine headaches.

Heroin. A chemically modified form of morphine with medical uses similar to those of morphine. Heroin is made from morphine in one chemical step. Heroin is illegal for medical use in the United States.

Meperidine (Demerol or Pethidine). A synthetic drug that produces effects similar to those of morphine, but that has markedly different chemical structure.

Methadone. A synthetic drug that differs in molecular structure from heroin or morphine. However, scientists believe the chemical structure of the essential active core of methadone is like that of the opiates.

Methadone is classified as a synthetic opiate. Its medical use is similar to that of morphine. Methadone is obtained through government license and is illegal for general medical use in the United States.

There are hundreds of other kinds of opiates – natural, chemically modified, or synthetic – that are not commonly used by addicts because they are not readily available, are expensive, are extremely dangerous, or give very unpleasant effects.

A report of the World Health Organization published by the United Nations in July 1972 states that annual medical needs for opiates are now met by 1,500 tons of opium, but at least 1,000 tons reach the illicit drug market.

Cocaine is classified with the opiates as a narcotic, but it is not really an opiate. It is a natural ingredient found in the coca plant and is often used in conjunction with opiates by addicts. Its primary medical uses are to relieve nasal congestion and as a local anesthetic.

Drug dose for pain relief

Table 13 indicates the amount of each of the opiates needed to achieve equal levels of pain relief. The duration of action for each is approximately four to five hours. Addicts in an escalating cycle of sensual abuse may use two and one-half times these doses, intravenously, five times per day. Dilaudid and heroin are clearly the most potent opiates.

Cost of maintenance and substitution therapy

Table 14 shows the cost of maintenance or substitution therapy for opiate addicts.

Table 13. *Amounts of various drugs needed for equal levels of pain relief*

Drug	Dose (milligrams)
Codeine	120.0
Demerol	90.0
Opium	100.0
Morphine	10.0
Methadone	9.0
Heroin	3.0
Dilaudid	1.5

Source: Adapted from Goodman and Gilman (1975).

Table 14. *Cost of opiate maintenance for addicts, 1972 (equivalent dose per person per day in dollars)*

	Opium (700 mg.)	Morphine (100 mg.)	Heroin (40 mg.)	Methadone (90 mg.)
United States				
Legal: prescription[a]	$34.00 retail	$1.30 retail	Not available	Not available
Legal: licensed centers[a]	$19.00 wholesale	$0.80 wholesale	Not available	Free or about $0.30
Illegal street price	$40.00 crude	$50.00[b]	$50.00[b]	$10.00–50.00[b]
Southeast Asia				
Kilo lots	$0.03[c]	$0.05[c]	$0.09[c]	
Small quantities	$0.10[c]		$0.13[c]	
England	Maintenance doses of opium, morphine, heroin, cocaine, or methadone plus sterile hypodermic equipment are dispensed to registered addicts at government clinics for about $0.30 per day.			

[a] Opium supplied as 58-ounce tincture of opium; morphine supplied as tablets for physicians.

[b] Morphine or methadone may be cut and sold as heroin at heroin prices. At least 15 percent of the street heroin in American cities is actually methadone sold at heroin prices.

[c] The price of opiates varied in Southeast Asia according to the quantity purchased and to the number of middle men in the chain of sellers. In 1971 and 1972, the average wholesale prices of opiates per gram in Saigon were: $2.25 (prices as low as $0.90 are reported – Candlin, 1973; Jones) for high grade heroin (#4, greater than 90 percent pure); $0.50 for morphine base; and $0.045 for raw opium. The retail price per gram for high grade heroin, sold in plastic vials each holding 300 milligrams of heroin, was $3.30 ($1.00 per plastic vial of 300 milligrams). With more middle men involved in the distribution, prices to soldiers were frequently as high as $12.00 per gram. (Sources: Candlin, 1973; Jones, personal observations made in Southeast Asia, 1971, 1972, and 1973; McCoy, 1972.)

Drug use among patients in treatment clinics

The figures presented here and in Chapter 5 are adapted from data given in *Summary of Client-Oriented Drug Abuse Information* prepared by the National Institute of Drug Abuse. The studies are based on 41,873 patients admitted to federally supported drug treatment centers in thirty-one cities in the United States between January 1, 1974, and March 31, 1975.

The data indicate a very rapid rise in admissions over the fifteen-month reporting period. The crude data indicate an increase of 13 percent per month in the total number of admissions. The increase in new cases only at treatment centers is 7 percent per month. This corresponds precisely to the rate of increase in drug abuse in the United States since the beginning of the drug movement in 1965. Those who have been severely affected by drugs have emerged from the much larger subpopulation of persons in the drug culture. The size of both groups is increasing at the same rate. Noting the rate of increase, it is possible to conclude that the number of drug users needing treatment will not reach a peak for several years.

The persons receiving treatment at the clinics had usually been part of the drug culture for several years prior to admission. In general, the interval between an individual's first drug experience and his first admission to a federal treatment clinic was 4.7 years for blacks, 4.2 years for people of Spanish descent, 3 years for whites, and 2.4 years for Asians or Indians.

Table 15 shows the status of the patients at discharge from the clinics during the study period. Of the patients admitted, for 55 percent opiate dependency was the primary problem. One-third of these were treated in methadone maintenance programs, and the remaining two-thirds were detoxified and treated by a drug-free regimen.

Table 15: *Status of patients at discharge from federally funded treatment clinics*

Status	Patients discharged (%)
Treatment incomplete	41.0
Treatment completed	21.3
Transferred to different method of treatment	23.5
Discharged for noncompliance	9.6
Incarcerated	4.2
Dead	0.4

Source: Data from U.S. National Institute of Drug Abuse (1975).

Some observable signs and symptoms of drug use

I have interviewed over 1,000 heavy drug users and have observed in them signs and symptoms of drug use. The list is long, and many of the signs and symptoms are the same. The discussion below is limited to a few I have observed to be particularly typical of each sensual drug.

Amphetamines. The chronic user often has acne resembling a measles rash. His hair is dry and lifeless. He may have gingivitis, caries, atrophy of the gums, and boils. If his drug use has induced brain damage, he may have difficulty in forming thoughts into words; his speech is slow, as if he were trying to speak a foreign language. The pupils of his eyes may be dilated, and in the acute stages of amphetamine use, the whites may be shiny.

Cocaine. Cocaine sniffing damages the nasal mucosa. The user may notice a dryness in his nose and mouth, followed by excessive nasal secretion, nosebleeds, and sloughing of the nasal mucosa. A hole may develop in his nasal septum. The chronic cocaine sniffer appears to have a runny cold. He may also have the same slow speech and dilated pupils as the amphetamine user. A toxic overdose of cocaine causes a decrease in the ability to taste or smell and a numbing of the mouth, nose, and teeth.

Alcohol. The staggering gait and slurred speech of the alcoholic are well known. The chronic user who drinks only small quantities may show no evidence of intoxication, but he will have traces of acetone and aldehydes on his breath; he will move at a slower pace; and the whites of his eyes may be yellowish from liver jaundice. After several decades of exposure to alcohol, the skin and connective tissue start to sag. When the alcoholic is not under the influence of alcohol, the enlarged vessels of the face are bluish; during periods of intoxication, the increased blood flow induced by alcohol causes these vessels to become red. The skin changes are most pronounced at the tip of the nose, which becomes bulbous and discolored.

Barbiturates. Barbiturate intoxication is similar to alcohol intoxication. Whereas the alcohol user may vomit, the barbiturate user usually does not; thus the barbiturate user absorbs more of the drug dose and may appear drunker. The barbiturate user can easily overdose. Typically, his speech is slurred; he walks unsteadily or staggers; he loses his balance easily and falls frequently. He may have more severe tremors than the alcoholic drunk; his hands, lips, and tongue tremble severely, and his eyes may roll. Barbiturates cannot be detected on the user's breath.

Opiates. The eyes of the opiate user are painfully sensitive to light, even after a fix when his pupils have constricted to pinpoints. Heroin addicts often wear dark glasses. Between fixes, eyes and pupils appear normal.

Before the urine test was developed, an eye pupil test was used to detect opiate use. The test consisted of giving an injection of naline, an opiate antagonist. The naline caused the pupils of the opiate user to enlarge noticeably within twenty minutes.

Another symptom of opiate addiction is the nodding and drowsiness that continue long after each fix.

Marijuana. Although it is often said that smoking marijuana a few times a month has no lasting effects, I have noticed that such an occasional user often has a pale complexion and diminished mobility of the vaso-motor coloration of the face. The chronic weekly user is unlikely to blush and the daily user cannot blush. During the period of cannabis intoxication, however, the skin becomes normal in color or even ruddy. The whites of the eyes, especially in the beginning user, may become red. The chronic daily user has little facial expression; it is as if his facial muscles are unable to change with his thoughts. The heavy marijuana smoker often has oscillatory secondary movements in his gait.

LSD. I have noted that those who have used LSD frequently have diffi-culty concentrating. They often have irregular eye movements during conversation; these occur when they are having flashbacks and their at-tention is briefly turned inward.

Tobacco. The chronic tobacco smoker tends to have reduced facial color owing to the decreased blood flow to the skin in his face. His skin has an aged look; his fingers and teeth are discolored; his senses of smell and taste are suppressed; and he coughs and shows other signs of irritated lungs and respiratory passages.

Rehabilitation of sexual functioning as an incentive to stop drug use

In my interviews with young drug users, I have found that those who were sexually mature before becoming addicted are more concerned about the loss of their capacity to function sexually than they are about any other sensory deprivation. Discussion about this loss and the potential for recovery is therefore a good way of motivating the addict to rehabilitate himself. This approach is particularly effective with "new" addicts.

The discussions I have had varied somewhat with each addict, but they seemed to follow a pattern. The material I have found useful to cover and the approaches I have found effective are discussed below.

1. The addict must be assured that the discussion will be kept confidential. It is usually best to talk with only one addict at a time. If groups are used, they must be kept small enough so that there can be a close relationship between the addict and the professional. I have had good results in the army with small discussion groups. If one drug user begins to talk freely about his problems, it opens the way for the others to follow.

2. The initial questions asked by the counselor should have nothing to do with sex.

3. The addict must be made to feel that the counselor knows what he is talking about, has a sincere interest in the addict, and is not judging him.

4. The adverse effects of drug use should be discussed, and any apparent effects in the addict should be noted. The addict should be led to the point where he makes these observations for himself. The counselor's questions should lead the addict to compare his present mental and physical condition with his condition before he started using drugs.

5. It should be explained to the addict that the main effects of the sensual drugs occur in the brain. The brain should be discussed as the "master control" of the body (see Chapter 2).

316

6. Only when the addict is ready should the discussion of his personal sexual problems begin. No one likes to admit sexual inadequacy, and the addict is even less likely to admit it than the nonaddict.

With opiate addicts, at this point I usually ask, "When did you first realize you were sexually incapacitated?" With women I ask when they became emotionally incapacitated. The reply is almost always, "When I began to use heroin." This direct approach avoids many layers of rationalization, and the admission is a breakthrough in the discussion. The way is then open for a frank discussion with the addict of his physical and emotional life before and after he became addicted.

With marijuana users, the approach is not so easy. The marijuana user is unable to have such direct insight into his sexual incapacitation. He is more confused and cannot notice changes in himself. I have found that a discussion with someone who is high on marijuana is ineffective in persuading him to abstain from marijuana use. The longer the time since the user's last exposure to marijuana, the easier it is to communicate with him.

Marijuana users often experience increased sexual activity early in their drug use; impotence comes later. Thus, the sexually incapacitated user often does not associate his sex problem with his use of the drug. The best way of dealing with this is to ask the user how recently he has had sexual dreams or how frequently he is involved in sexual activity, including masturbation. Regular dreaming and the ability to remember dreams are suppressed in the marijuana user. The counselor's questions may reveal this to him.

Self-testing is the most effective way for a marijuana user to recognize his sexual incapacity. I have interviewed many young men who claimed they had not experienced any sexual difficulties as a result of marijuana use, but who, after six weeks of abstinence, noticed a recovery of sexual capacity they did not realize they had lost.

Sensual drugs can cause a general reduction in sexual capacity and desire or more specific disturbances, such as lack of sexual dreaming, premature or delayed ejaculation, prolonged erection, delayed orgasm, or inability to reach orgasm. Getting the addict to recognize these disturbances as drug-related is important. The purpose of asking the addict questions about his earlier sexual experiences is not to make him share intimate details, but to enable him to recall his sexual capacity before he became dependent on drugs.

7. The counselor should explain to the addict that his sexual incapacity is just one manifestation of the sensory deprivation that has taken place. The degree of sexual deprivation is a good measure of how much other sensory functions may be suppressed. The addict's inability to sleep

soundly, his lapses in memory, and his difficulty in concentrating should be discussed. The addict is usually unable to have close relationships; he often blames others (or society) for his problems. He must be helped toward an understanding of how these problems are caused or aggravated by his drug use.

8. The addict has to want to return to his drug-free state more than he wants drugs. He should be reassured that his sexual and other disturbed functions can return to normal if he abstains from using sensual drugs. He should be made to feel that he can break his drug habit, that he has a choice.

9. The first session is often the best time to uncover the addict's rationalizations about his drug use. His insights about his sexual functioning are often the jolt he needs to give up drugs. No matter how willing he may be to try a drug-free life, his resolve must be strengthened every day. The counselor should explain that the return of his brain's mechanisms to normal takes time, that the rate of recovery varies from addict to addict, and that he will have to wait for noticeable results.

Even if the addict does not resolve to end his drug use immediately, a discussion such as the one outlined above makes him look carefully at what drugs have done to him. The limitations of this approach are that the addict must have begun to use drugs after reaching sexual maturity and that he must not have severe emotional disturbances.

U.S. Senate hearings on world drug traffic

Because of the threat to the internal security of the United States, the Internal Security Subcommittee of the Senate Committee on the Judiciary in 1972 and 1973 held hearings that focused on the world drug traffic. Although little publicized, these hearings are an excellent source of information on the drug problem.

The hearings covered the following subjects:

1972   Part I (August 14): Drug traffic in Southeast Asia
1972   Part II (September 12): The hashish trail
1972   Part III (September 13 and 15): The international connection
1972   Part IV (September 14): Drug traffic – the global context
1972   Part V (September 18): Research on marijuana and hashish
1973   (October 3): Hashish smuggling and passport fraud

U.S. Senate hearings on marijuana and hashish

After the Senate hearings on world drug traffic in 1972 and 1973 (Appendix 7), the Subcommittee on Internal Security of the Senate Committee on the Judiciary decided to look into the marijuana-hashish epidemic in the United States. Dr. O. J. Braenden, Director of the U.N. Narcotics Laboratory, Geneva, was especially persuasive in pointing out the need for more extensive hearings on the recent scientific evidence of the dangers of cannabis drug use.

The 1974 hearings focused on the scientific evidence for the physical and psychological effects of cannabis. Scientists and experts in various fields from all over the world were invited to testify. These hearings present the most comprehensive collection of scientific evidence yet published on the harmful effects of marijuana. The hearings in 1975 set forth evidence on the escalation of the potency and quantity of cannabis drugs used in the United States.

Following is a list of scientific and other expert witnesses who appeared before the subcommittee:

Scientific witnesses, 1974 hearings

Julius Axelrod: chemist, pharmacologist. Awarded the Nobel Prize in physiology and medicine in 1970 for study of drug effects on the brain; Chief, Section on Pharmacology, National Institute of Mental Health

Nils Bejerot: physician, psychiatrist, epidemiologist. Karolinska Institute, Sweden; author of *Addiction and Society* and several standard texts on the epidemiology of drug abuse; widely recognized as one of the foremost international experts in this field

Henry Brill: physician, psychiatrist. Regional Director, New York State Department of Mental Hygiene; member and/or chairman of drug dependence committees of the American Medical Association, the National Research Council, the World Health Organization, and the Food and Drug Administration; senior psychiatric member of the Shafer Commission

John A.S. Hall: Senior Physician and Chairman, Department of Medicine, Kingston Hospital, Jamaica (since 1965); Associate Lecturer in Medicine, University of West Indies; Visiting Assistant Professor of Neurology, Columbia University

Robert Heath: physician, psychiatrist, neurologist. Professor and Chairman, Department of Psychiatry and Neurology, Tulane University Medical School

Hardin B. Jones: physiologist, biophysicist, epidemiologist. Professor of Physiology and Professor of Medical Physics, University of California, Berkeley; Assistant Director, Donner Laboratory of Medical Physics, Berkeley

Harold Kolansky: physician, psychiatrist. Professor of Psychiatry, University of Pennsylvania School of Medicine; twice President, Regional Council (Pennsylvania, New Jersey, Delaware) of Child Psychiatry; Director of Child Psychiatry, Albert Einstein Medical Center, Philadelphia (1955–1969); Chairman, Department of Psychiatry, Albert Einstein Medical Center (1968–1969)

Robert Kolodny: physician, endocrinologist. Director, Endocrine Research Section, Reproductive Biology Research Foundation, Saint Louis

Cecile Leuchtenberger: cytologist, biophysicist. Head, Department of Cell Chemistry, Institute for Experimental Cancer Research, Lausanne, Switzerland; founder and first director, Cell Chemistry Department, Western Reserve University

Donald Louria: physician, epidemiologist. Chairman, Department of Preventive Medicine and Community Health, New Jersey Medical School; Chairman and President, New York State Council on Drug Addiction (to 1972)

Andrew Malcolm: physician, psychiatrist. Member, Drug Advisory Committee, Ontario College of Pharmacy; Senior Psychiatrist, Rockland State Hospital, New York (1955–1958)

William T. Moore: physician, psychiatrist. Professor in Clinical Psychiatry, University of Pennsylvania School of Medicine; Professor of Child Psychiatry, Hahnemann Medical College (for thirteen years until 1972); Director of Training, Division of Child Analysis, Institute of Philadelphia Association for Psychoanalysis (1971–)

Akira Morishima: physician, pediatrician, geneticist. Professor, Department of Pediatrics, Columbia University College of Physicians and Surgeons; Chief, Division of Pediatric Endocrine Service, Babies Hospital, New York

Gabriel Nahas: physician, physiologist, immunologist. Professor, Columbia University College of Physicians and Surgeons; Adjunct Professor, University of Paris, Faculty of Medicine

W. D. M. Paton: physician, pharmacologist, pathologist, physiologist. Head, Department of Pharmacology, Oxford University; chairman of committee overseeing the British government's drug research program; author of standard textbook on pharmacology and widely recognized as one of the world's leading pharmacologists

Harvey Powelson: physician, psychiatrist. Clinical psychiatrist, University of California Medical School, San Francisco, and Chief, Psychiatric Division, Student Health Services, University of California, Berkeley (1964–1972)

Conrad Schwarz: physician, psychiatrist. Professor, Department of Psychiatry, University of British Columbia; Consultant Psychiatrist, Student Health Service, University of British Columbia; Chairman, Drug Habituation Committee, British Columbia Medical Association.

M. I. Soueif: physiologist. Chairman, Department of Psychology and Philosophy, Cairo University; member, World Health Organization Panel on Drug Dependence; author of classic study on the consequences of hashish addiction in Egypt

Morton Stenchever: physician, obstetrician, gynecologist, cytogeneticist. Chairman, Department of Obstetrics and Gynecology, University of Utah Medical School

Forest S. Tennant, Jr.: physician, drug abuse specialist. Medical director for several drug abuse programs in the Los Angeles area; officer in charge of the drug abuse program of the U.S. Army in Europe (1971–1972)

Phillip Zeidenberg: physician, psychiatrist, specialist in drug abuse. Professor of Psychiatry, Columbia University; Chairman, Drug Dependence Committee, New York State Psychiatric Institute

Arthur M. Zimmerman: Professor of Zoology, University of Toronto, Toronto, Canada

Other expert witnesses, 1974 hearings

Frank B. Clay: Major General, U.S. Army. Deputy Assistant Secretary of Defense, Drug and Alcohol Abuse

David O. Cooke: Deputy Assistant Secretary of Defense; accompanied by Dr. John F. Mazzuchi, Brig. Gen. W. A. Temple, Col. Frank W.

Zimmerman, David N. Planton, Comdr. S. J. Kreider, Col. Henry H. Tufts, Col. Wayne B. Sargent, and Col. John J. Castellot

Keith Cowan: advisor to Canadian government in province of Prince Edward Island; director of an institute associated with the University of Prince Edward Island; member, Public Drug Education Committee, Department of Education

Andrew C. Tartaglino: Acting Deputy Administrator, Drug Enforcement Administration

Witnesses, 1975 hearings

Robert L. DuPont: physician, psychiatrist. Director, Special Action Office for Drug Abuse Prevention; Director, National Institute on Drug Abuse; Clinical Professor of Psychiatry and Behavioral Science, George Washington University School of Medicine

Jerry N. Jenson: Deputy Administrator, Drug Enforcement Administration, Department of Justice; accompanied by Robert I. Rosthal, Depute Chief Counsel

Carlton E. Turner: chemist, pharmacologist. Director, Marihuana Project, School of Pharmacy, University of Mississippi

Coy W. Waller: chemist, pharmacologist. Director, Research Institute of Pharmaceutical Sciences and Professor of Pharmaceutics, University of Mississippi; formerly vice president in charge of research, Meade-Johnson Company

THC: two animal studies

Physiological effects of THC on rats

Rosenkrantz and Luthra and their colleagues (1975) have done one of the more extensive studies to date on the physiological effects of marijuana.

Groups of male and female rats were given oral doses of 2, 10, or 50 milligrams of THC per kilogram of body weight for 28, 90, and 180 days. Another group of rats, treated for 180 days, was studied after a 30-day recovery period. The lowest dose used in the study, adjusted for differences in metabolic rate between species (see under "Relation of animal and human studies," Chapter 10), corresponded to the THC dose for humans of one high-grade marijuana cigarette; the intermediate dose corresponded to the THC content of one hashish cigarette.

During the first 10 days on THC, the rats showed lack of coordination, ataxia, passivity, slowed breathing, and difficulty in regulating body temperature. During the next 10 to 20 days, they were irritable, hypersensitive, hyperactive, and aggressive. Fighting, tremors, and convulsions occurred among the animals given the higher doses. These effects abated with time, showing that tolerance to the dose had developed.

At autopsy, forty-nine physiological measurements were made on each of the 192 rats in the study. The researchers found dramatic shifts in water balance, changes in the brain enzymes, and a decrease in RNA in the cerebral hemispheres. Blood sugar levels increased significantly even at the lowest dose of THC and in the shortest period of observation. This disturbance continued, even at the lowest level of exposure, for a month after the THC was withdrawn from the rats. In spite of increased food consumption, growth decreased. There was a marked dose-related decrease in water intake. Although body weight decreased, most organ weights increased.

The increase in organ weight varied considerably, but the variations largely disappeared upon cessation of exposure to THC. This suggests that the increase in organ weight (including the brain) was due to edema (fluid retention). In male rats, the prostate decreased in weight – a possible indication of hormonal disturbances.

Some of the dose-related effects were the same in both male and female rats; other effects were different in males and females. Acetylcholinesterase, a brain enzyme, was elevated in the male rats and decreased in the females. In some instances, the declines in RNA and proteins were sex-related. Further analysis of the data showed that during the recovery period the brain weight of the male rats returned to that of the controls, but the females' brain weight increased on all doses of THC to levels higher than those of the controls. The wide range of systematic differences between males and females leads to the conclusion that THC has a varied pattern of influence on centers of physiologic controls and on brain chemistry.

The experimenters concluded: "It has been demonstrated that chronic treatment with reasonable doses of delta-9-THC introduces neurochemical and neurotoxicological manifestations. Several of these occurred after tolerance, which implies some form of cumulative toxicity. Not all neurochemical abnormalities are reversible after 30 days of recovery" (Luthra *et al.*, 1975).

Effects of THC on monkey brains

Heath has completed a definitive study showing that marijuana causes brain atrophy, synaptic changes, and pronounced effects in EEG recordings from the limbic structures in monkeys (Heath, 1973; U.S. Senate Hearings, 1974; 1976, personal communication).

Thirteen rhesus monkeys were used in the study. Minute electrodes were permanently implanted deep in the brains of ten monkeys – in the septal region, the hippocampus, the amygdala (see Figure 2), the sensory relay centers, and the centers where cells are known to be activated by specific chemical transmitters. Three monkeys were left intact to act as controls. Scalp recordings and electrocardiograms were always obtained on the thirteen monkeys.

A special apparatus permitted delivery of marijuana smoke of precisely measured amounts of THC to the monkeys. Each monkey was exposed to a predetermined dose of THC for six months as follows:

Heavy smokers: three times a day, five days a week. Adjusted for differences in metabolic rate between species (see under "Relation of animal and human studies," Chapter 10), this is equivalent to seven joints of marijuana per day for humans, based on a joint of 1.5 grams of 3 percent Δ-9-THC.

Moderate smokers: two times a week with the dose per smoke the same as for the heavy smoking monkeys. This is equivalent to one joint per day for humans.

Light smokers: exposed to one-half the smoke of the moderate smokers. This is equivalent to one-half joint per day for humans.

Monkeys injected with THC: two monkeys were given THC intravenously in doses that would simulate the behavior and immediate EEG changes caused by the heavy and moderate doses given to the THC-smoking monkeys.

Monkeys not exposed to THC: two monkeys smoked inactive marijuana three times a day, five days a week – the same schedule that was used for the heavy smokers.

The heavy and moderate doses induced distinct, acute changes in behavior. The monkeys responded less to all forms of sensory stimuli (pin pricks, hand clapping, etc.), stared blankly into space, and displayed slowed motor movement.

Deep and surface electrode recordings in the moderate and heavy smokers showed distinct changes in many brain regions, but they were most consistent in the septal region, the hippocampus, and the amygdala. When the monkeys displayed catatonic behavior, the recordings resembled those the researchers had previously obtained from the septal region of severely disturbed psychotic patients. At other times, when the monkeys behaved as if they might be hallucinating, recording changes were most pronounced in the sensory relay centers, and recordings from the centers of brain cells having specific transmitter chemicals were also affected.

Changes in the recordings of the two monkeys who received THC injections were similar to, but more pronounced than, those obtained from monkeys exposed to the smoke of active marijuana. On injection, the changes occurred within one minute. In the smoking monkeys, the behavior and recording changes came on gradually and were quite pronounced at the end of the five-minute exposure. There was a gradual return to base line in thirty to forty minutes.

These acute behavior and recording effects were not seen in the light smokers or in the heavy smokers of inactive marijuana.

Changes in scalp recordings were not significant. When they did occur, they were nonspecific and reflected alterations in levels of awareness, such as drowsiness.

As time passed, chronic changes in brain activity occurred; the septal region, the hippocampus, and the amygdala were the most profoundly affected. In the moderate and heavy smokers, the persistent brain wave changes became apparent in about three months. The persistent brain wave changes in the injected monkeys were evident in two to three months.

Two of the heavy smokers died of respiratory complications during the study, one three and one-half months and the other five and one-half months after the study had begun. The histopathologic report on the brains indicated that minimal structural changes had occurred in the cells of the septal region.

The monkeys were observed for eight months following the six-month exposure period. In the monkeys exposed to THC through smoke and by injection, EEG alterations from the deep brain sites persisted unchanged through the entire eight-month postexposure period. The two monkeys exposed to inactive marijuana continued to have normal readings.

At the end of the eight-month postexposure period, the monkeys were sacrificed. Their brains were immediately preserved before cell changes could take place so that they could be submitted to anatomical and histological studies. Under an ordinary light microscope, no changes were detectable in the brains; under an electron microscope, changes were detected in the brains that correlated with the deep brain EEG readings. These changes occurred in monkeys given moderate and high doses and in those exposed to THC by smoking or by injection. In the septal region, distinct changes in the synapses occurred: a significant widening of the synaptic cleft, an accumulation of radiopaque material, and a clumping of the synaptic vesicles – an early sign of neuronal degeneration. The ventricles were enlarged, indicating that the subcortical areas (containing the limbic structures) proximal to the ventricles had atrophied. This important observation confirms the findings of Campbell *et al.* (1971) of cerebral atrophy in young heavy marijuana smokers.

The brains of the control monkeys, which were not exposed to THC, and of the monkeys which had been light smokers showed no abnormal changes. Because the monkeys were exposed to THC for only six months, the time was too short for observable changes to develop in the brains of the light smokers.

As this book goes to press, Heath's findings on the changes in the synapses and ventricles in the brains of monkeys exposed to THC have been submitted for publication. It will take months and perhaps years of laboratory work to study the myriad nerve tracts of each brain and to determine the number of brain cells that have been affected.

Cannabis seizures

The alarming increase in the use of cannabis drugs in the United States is reflected in seizures of illicit marijuana (Table 16). Officials estimate that only 10 to 20 percent of the illicit shipments of marijuana are seized.

The more recent seizures have been of higher grades of marijuana. Before 1970, the marijuana grown in the United States was a very weak variety with an average THC content of about 0.2 percent. Since 1970, more potent Mexican varieties have been imported to the United States in greater quantities. Marijuana seized by authorities between 1971 and 1974 averaged about 1.92 percent THC. Since 1974, marijuana seized in the United States has typically had a THC content of 3 to 4 percent, and some, usually grown in Central and South America, has had a THC content of 14 percent.

Table 16. *Increase in United States government seizures of marijuana, 1969–1974*

Year	Total seized (kg.)	Increase over previous year (kg.)	Annual increase in seizures (%)
1969	29,500		
1970	83,500	54,000	183
1971	135,200	51,700	62
1972	229,900	94,700	70
1973	349,300	119,400	52
1974	911,300	562,000	161

Source: U.S. Senate hearings (1975).

Seizures of hashish oil are also increasing. In 1970, 2,800 kilograms were seized by federal authorities; in 1974, 23,000 kilograms were seized. This is an increase of 820 percent over a four-year period, or 105 percent per year. Much more hashish oil is probably consumed in the United States than these figures indicate, for the percentage of hashish oil intercepted is probably much lower than the percentage of marijuana seized. The concentrated form is more easily smuggled.

Seizures of hashish have not increased as rapidly. From 1973 to 1974, the increase was 10 percent, compared with the 161 percent for marijuana and the 105 percent for hashish oil. This slowdown can be explained partly by the availability of high-potency marijuana. Hashish from the Middle East has been limited to about 10 percent THC because, until recently, it was produced only as a by-product of the hemp industry. The strains of hemp grown in Central and South America for the illicit market contain a much higher percentage of THC. If labor becomes available for harvesting hashish resin in addition to the leaves and flowers of this potent variety, we may expect to see an increase in the amounts of the stronger grades of hashish smuggled into the United States. (See U.S. Senate Hearings, 1975, for more information on the increase of cannabis consumption in the United States.)

Mortality rate and drug abuse

For many years there has been a steady annual decline in the mortality rate. In the mid-1960s this trend reversed abruptly in the United States in the male population between fifteen and thirty-five years of age. The total death risk in this subpopulation increased approximately 30 percent between 1961 and 1971 – from 1.0 to 1.3 deaths per 1,000 yearly. In 1971 (latest available data) there was an increase of about 12,000 deaths over the deaths recorded in a comparable population in 1961. Motor vehicle accidents were responsible for a significant portion of the increase (Table 17).

Links between the rise in mortality rate and drug abuse are shown in several ways: (1) the coincidence of the increased mortality with the beginning of the drug abuse epidemic, (2) the steady increase in drug use and the death rate since 1965, and (3) the greater rise in both mortality rate and drug abuse in the male population. The rise in drug abuse and in death risk first occurred among the college-aged population; in later calendar years younger and older ages were also affected.

Table 17. *Percent increase in accidental deaths in total United States population, 1961–1971, by age of victim*

Type of accident	Age of victim (years)			
	15–19	20–24	25–29	30–34
All accidents	35	26	19	24
Motor vehicle accidents	41	27	22	26

Bibliography

Bibliography

Abel, E. L. 1971. Marijuana and memory: Acquisition or retrieval. *Science* 173:1038–1040.

Abrahamsen, D. 1958. *The Road to Emotional Maturity*. Englewood Cliffs, N.J.: Prentice-Hall.

Agurell, S., *et al*. 1972. Metabolic fate of tetrahydrocannabinol. In *Cannabis and Its Derivatives*, edited by W. D. M. Paton and J. Crown. London: Oxford University Press.

Altman, L. 1973. Swedes develop marijuana test. *New York Times*, July 12, p. 15.

A.M.A. Committee on Alcoholism and Addiction. 1965. Dependence on barbiturates and other sedative drugs. *J.A.M.A.* 193:673–677.

Ames, F. A. 1958. A clinical and metabolic study of acute intoxication with "cannabis sativa" and its role in the model psychoses. *J. Ment. Sci.* 104:972–999.

Angrist, B., and Gershon, S. 1972. Some recent studies in amphetamine psychosis: Unresolved issues. In *Current Concepts on Amphetamine Abuse*, edited by E. H. Ellinwood and S. Cohen. Proceedings of a workshop, Duke University Medical Center, June 5–6, 1970. Washington: G.P.O.

Appel, J. B., and Freedman, D. X. 1965. The relative potencies of psychotomimetic drugs. *Life Sci.* 4:2181–2186.

Asimov, I. 1964. *The Human Brain: Its Capacities and Functions*. Boston: Houghton Mifflin.

Ausubel, D. P. 1960. Controversial issues in the management of drug addiction: Legalization, ambulatory treatment and the British system. *Ment. Hyg.* 44:535–544.

Axelrod, J., *et al*. 1971. Findings reported on analysis of the metabolic fate of delta-9-THC. *Pharmacol. Rev.* 23:371–380.

Baden, M. M. 1971. Methadone related deaths in New York City. *Int. J. Addict.* 5:489–498.

Balter, M. B. 1968. The use of drugs in contemporary society. *Highlights, 14th Annual Conference, Veterans Administration Cooperative Studies in Psychiatry, April 1, 1968.* Washington: Veterans Administration.

Balter, M. B., and Levine, J. 1971. Character and extent of psychotherapeutic drug usage in the United States. Paper presented at the 5th World Congress on Psychiatry, November 30, 1971, Mexico City.

Bass, M. 1970. Sudden sniffing death. *J.A.M.A.* 212:2075–2079.

Bazell, R. J. 1973. Drug abuse: Methadone becomes the solution and the problem. *Science* 179:772–775.

Beaubrun, M. H. 1973. Drug abuse in different cultural groups in Jamaica. *Jamaican Psychiatr. News*, December 19, p. 9.

Beaubrun, M. H., and Knight, F. 1973. Psychiatric assessment of thirty chronic users of cannabis and thirty matched controls. *Am. J. Psychiatry* 130:309–311.

Bejerot, N. 1970*a*. *Addiction and Society*. Springfield, Ill. Thomas.
    1970*b*. A comparison of the effects of cocaine and synthetic central stimulants. *Br. J. Addict.* 65:35–37.

Bell, D. S., and Trethowan, W. H. 1961. Amphetamine addiction and disturbed sexuality. *Arch. Gen. Psychiatry* 4:74–78.

Benabud, A. 1957. Psycho-pathological aspects of the cannabis situation in Morocco. *Bull. Narc. (U.N.)* 9 (4):1–16.

Bensusan, A. D. 1971. Marihuana withdrawal symptoms. *Br. Med. J.* 3:112.

Bewley, T. 1965. Heroin and cocaine addiction. *Lancet* 1:808–810.

Birnell, J. H. W. 1971. Some aspects of alcohol and road collisions. In *Alcoholism and Drug Dependency*, edited by L. G. Kiloh and D. S. Bell. London: Butterworth.

Black, P. (ed.). 1969. *Drugs and the Brain*. Baltimore: Johns Hopkins Press.

Bleuler, E. 1950. *Dementia Praecox or the Group of Schizophrenias*. New York: International Universities Press.

Blevins, R. D., and Regan, J. D. 1976. Delta-9-tetrahydrocannabinol: Effect on macromolecular synthesis in human and other mammalian cells. In *Marihuana: Chemistry, Biochemistry, and Cellular Effects*, edited by G. G. Nahas *et al*. New York: Springer-Verlag.

Blumberg, H. H. 1975. Surveys of drug use among young people. *Int. J. Addict.* 10:699–719.

Bohus, B., and de Wied, D. 1966. Inhibitory and facilitatory effect of two related peptides on extinction of avoidance behavior. *Science* 153:318–320.

Brill, H. 1970. Pro-drug dialectic communication on drug abuse and the marijuana red herring. In *Communication and Drug Abuse*, edited by J. R. Wittenborn *et al.* Springfield, Ill.: Thomas.

Brill, H., and Hirose, T. 1969. The rise and fall of the methamphetamine epidemic: Japan 1945–1955. *Semin. Psychiatry* 1:179–194.

Brill, L., and Harms, E. 1972. *Yearbook of Drug Abuse.* New York: Behavioral Publications.

Brill, N. Q., and Christie, R. L. 1974. Marihuana use and psychosocial adaptation: Follow-up study of a collegiate population. *Arch. Gen. Psychiatry* 31:713–731.

Brill, N. Q , *et al.* 1970. The marijuana problem: UCLA interdepartmental conference. *Ann. Int. Med.* 73:449–465.

Brown, B. B. 1968. Some characteristic EEG differences between heavy smoker and nonsmoker subjects. *Neuropsychologia* 6:381–388.

    1974. *New Mind, New Body.* New York: Harper & Row.

Burford, R., *et al.* 1975. The combined effects of alcohol and common psychoactive drugs. 1. Studies on human pursuit tracking capability. In *Alcohol, Drugs, and Traffic Safety: Proceedings of the 6th International Conference on Alcohol, Drugs, and Traffic Safety, Toronto, September 8–13, 1974*, edited by S. Israelstam and S. Lambert. Toronto: Addiction Research Foundation of Ontario.

Byrd, O. E. (ed.). 1970. *Medical Readings on Drug Abuse.* Reading Mass.: Addision-Wesley.

Caldwell, J., and Sever, P. S. 1974. The biochemical pharmacology of abused drugs. *Clin. Pharmacol. Ther.* 16:625–638.

Campbell, A. M. G., *et al.* 1971. Cerebral atrophy in young cannabis smokers. *Lancet* 2:1219–1224.

Campbell, D.R. 1971. The electroencephalogram in cannabis associated psychosis. *Can. Psychiatr. Assoc. J.* 16:161–165.

Campbell, H. J. 1971. Pleasure-seeking brains: Artificial tickles, natural joys of thought. *Smithsonian* 2(7):14–23.

Campbell, R. 1971. The brain. IV. Chemistry of madness. *Life*, November 26, pp. 66–86.

Canada Commission of Inquiry into the Non-Medical Use of Drugs. 1970. *Interim Report of the Commission . . . .* Ottawa: Information Canada.

    1972. *Treatment: A report of the Commission . . . .* Ottawa: Information Canada.

1972. *Cannabis: A report of the Commission* . . . . Ottawa: Information Canada.

1973. *Final Report of the Commission* . . . . Ottawa: Information Canada.

Candlin, A. H. S. 1973. *Psychochemical Warfare*. New Rochelle: Arlington House.

Chambers, C. D., and Taylor, W. R. 1970. Patterns of "cheating" among methadone maintenance patients. Paper presented at the Eastern Psychiatric Research Association Meeting, November 7, 1970, New York.

Chapin, W. 1972. *Wasted: The Story of My Son's Drug Addiction*. New York: McGraw-Hill.

Chessick, R. D. 1960. The pharmacogenic orgasm in the drug addict. *Arch. Gen. Psychiatry* 3:545–556

Chopra, G. S. 1971. Marijuana and adverse psychotic reactions. *Bull. Narc. (U.N.)* 23(3):15–22.

Chopra, G. S., and Smith, J. W. 1974. Psychotic reactions following cannabis use in East Indies. *Arch. Gen. Psychiatry* 30:24–27.

Chopra, R. N., and Chopra, G. S. 1939. The present position of hemp-drug addiction in India. *Indian J. Med. Res. Memoir* 31:1–119 (supplementary series).

Chopra, R. N., and Chopra, I. C. 1965. *Drug Addiction with Special Reference to India*. New York: International Publications Service.

Cicero, T. J., *et al*. 1975. Function of the male sex organs in heroin and methadone users. *N. Engl. J. Med.* 292:882–887.

Clark, L. D., *et al*. 1970. Behavioral effects of marihuana: Experimental studies. *Arch. Gen. Psychiatry* 33:193–198.

Clouet, D. H. (ed.). 1971. *Narcotic Drugs: Biochemical Pharmacology*. New York: Plenum Press.

Cohen, M. M., *et al*. 1967. Chromosomal damage in human leukocytes induced by lysergic acid diethylamide. *Science* 155:1417–1419.

Cohen, S. 1966. A classification of LSD complications. *Psychosomatics* 7:182–186.

1975. Glue sniffing. *J.A.M.A.* 231:653–654.

Collier, H. O. 1972. The experimental analysis of drug dependence. *Endeavor* 31(114):123–129.

Collier, H. O., *et al*. 1972. Modification of morphine withdrawal by drugs interacting with humoral mechanisms: Some contradictions and their interpretation. *Nature* 237:220–223.

Connell, P. H. 1964. Amphetamine misuse. *Br. J. Addict.* 60:9–27.

Cooper, D. L. 1972. Drugs and the Athlete. *J.A.M.A.* 221:1007–1011.

Cox, B. M., *et al*. 1975. A peptide-like substance from pituitary that acts like morphine: Purification and properties. *Life Sci.* 16:1777–1782.

Crowley, A. 1972. *The Diary of a Drug Fiend*. New York: Lancer Books.

Davis, J. 1970. Marijuana and driving performance. Audiotape transcribed in A *Drug Is Guilty Until Proven Innocent*, statement presented to the Commission of Inquiry into the Non-Medical Use of Drugs, directed by J. E. Blanchard and G. Bennett, November 6, 1970, Charlottetown, Prince Edward Island, Canada.

de Alarcón, R. 1969. The spread of heroin abuse in a community. *Bull. Narc.* (*U.N.*) 21(3):17–22.

De Leon, G., and Wexler, H. K. 1973. Heroin addiction: Its relation to sexual behavior and sexual experience. *J. Abnorm. Psychol.* 81:36–38.

Delgado, J. 1975. Exploring inner space. *Saturday Review*, August 9, pp. 21–25.

De Long, J. V. 1975. The methadone habit. *New York Times Magazine*, March 16, p. 16.

Dennen, A. 1971. Cerebral hemorrhage due to stimulants. *Med. J. Aust.* 2:101–102.

DeRopp, R. 1957. *Drugs and the Mind*. New York: Grove Press.
  1969. *Sex Energy*. New York: Delacorte Press.

de Wied, D., and Bohus, B. 1966. Long-term and short-term effects on retention of a conditioned avoidance response in rats by treatment with long-acting pitressin and α-MSH. *Science* 153:1484–1486.

Dimbley, J. 1971. The wide-open British drug scene. *New Republic* 164:15–16.

Dobbs, W. H. 1971. Methadone treatment of heroin addicts. *J.A.M.A.* 218:1536–1541.

Dole, V. P., and Nyswander, M. 1965. A medical treatment for diacetylmorphine (heroin) addiction: A clinical trial with methadone hydrochloride. *J.A.M.A.* 193:646–650.

Drachman, D. A., and Hughes, J. R. 1971. Memory and the hippocampal complexes. III. Aging and temporal EEG abnormalities. *Neurology* 21(1):1–14.

Eccles, J. 1965. The synapse. *Sci. Am.* 212(1):56–66.

Edwards, G. 1975. Marihuana. *Nature* 254:541.

Einstein, S. 1970. *The Use and Misuse of Drugs*. Basic Concepts in Health Series. Belmont, Cal.: Wadsworth.

Endore, G. 1967. *Synanon*. Garden City, N.Y.: Doubleday.

Epstein, E. J. 1974. Methadone: The forlorn hope. *Public Interest* 36:3–24.

Essig, C. F. 1966. Newer sedative drugs that can cause states of intoxication and dependence of barbiturate type. *J.A.M.A.* 196:714–716.

Evans, M. 1974. Cannabis and cerebral atrophy. *R. Soc. Health J.* 94:15–18.

Ewing, J. A., and Bakewell, W. E. 1967. Diagnosis and management of depressant drug dependence. *Am. J. Psychiatry* 123:909–917.

Fairbairn, J. W. 1974. Cannabinoid content of some English reefers. *Nature* 249:276–278.

Feldberg, W. 1963. *A Pharmacological Approach to the Brain from Its Inner and Outer Surface.* Baltimore: Williams & Wilkins.

Ferguson, P., *et al.* (eds.). 1974. *Drugs and Pregnancy: The Nonmedical Use of Drugs and Sexual Behavior.* Research Issues Series, No. 5. Prepared for the National Institute on Drug Abuse by Documentation Associates, Los Angeles. U.S. Department of Health, Education, and Welfare Publication No. (ADM)75–187 (printed 1975).

    1974. *Drugs and Sex: The Nonmedical Use of Drugs and Sexual Behavior.* Research Issues Series, No. 2. Prepared for the National Institute on Drug Abuse by Documentation Associates, Los Angeles. U.S. Department of Health, Education, and Welfare Publication No. (ADM)75–184 (printed 1975).

Fisher, A. 1975. The real dope on pot: New test suggest marijuana may have harmful effects. In *Nature Science Annual Edition.* New York: Time-Life Books.

Ford Foundation. 1972. *Dealing with Drug Abuse.* Report to the Ford Foundation. New York: Praeger.

Forney, R. B. 1971. Toxicology of marihuana. *Pharmacol. Rev.* 23:279–284.

Frohman, L. A. 1975. Neurotransmitters as regulators of endocrine function. *Hosp. Practice* 10(4):54–67.

Frosch, W. A., *et al.* 1965. Untoward reactions to lysergic acid diethylamide (LSD) resulting in hospitalization. *N. Engl. J. Med.* 273:1235–1239.

Fudge, J. W., and Penk, W. E. 1973. Methadone treatment and drug experimentation. *Science* 181:702.

Galin, D., and Ornstein, R. 1975. Hemispheric specialization and the duality of consciousness. In *Human Behavior and Brain Function,* edited by H. J. Widroe. Springfield, Ill.: Thomas.

Gardner, H. 1975. Brain damage: A window on the mind. *Saturday Review,* August 9, pp. 26–29.

Gary, N. E., and Keylon, V. 1970. Intravenous administration of marihuana. *J.A.M.A.* 211:501.

Gay, G. R., and Sheppard, C. W. 1973. Sex-crazed dope fiends: Myth or reality? In *Drugs and Youth: The Challenge of Today*, edited by E. Harms. New York: Pergamon Press.

Gellhorn, E., and Loofbourrow, G. N. 1963. *Emotions and Emotional Disorders: A Neurophysiological Study*. New York: Harper & Row.

Gill, E. W., and Jones, G. 1972. Brain levels of delta-1-tetrahydrocannabinol and its metabolites in mice: Correlation with behavior and the effect of the metabolic inhibitors SKF 525A and piperonyl butoxide. *Biochem. Pharmacol.* 21:2237–2248.

Gill, E. W., *et al.* 1972. Chemical mechanisms of action of THC. In *Cannabis and Its Derivatives*, edited by W. D. M. Paton and J. Crown. London: Oxford University Press.

   1973. Contributions of the metabolic 7-hydroxy-delta-1-tetrahydrocannabinol towards the pharmacological activity of delta-1-tetrahydrocannabinol in mice. *Biochem. Pharmacol.* 22:175–184.

Gilmour, D. G., *et al.* 1971. Chromosomal aberrations in users of psychoactive drugs. *Arch. Gen. Psychiatry* 24:268–272.

Glass, L., and Evans, H. E. 1972. Narcotic withdrawal in the newborn. *Am. Fam. Physician* 6(1):75–78.

Glatt, M. M., *et al.* 1967. *The Drug Scene in Great Britain*. London: Edward Arnold.

Gombrich, E. H. 1972. The visual image. *Sci. Am.* 227(3):82–96.

Goode, E. 1969. Marijuana and sex. *Evergreen Rev.* 66:19.

   1972. Drug use and sexual activity on a college campus. *Am. J. Psychiatry* 128:1272–1276.

Goodman, L., and Gilman, A. (eds.). 1975. *The Pharmacological Basis of Therapeutics*, 5th ed. New York: Macmillan.

Gore, R., *et al.* 1971. The brain. III. The mind in action. *Life*, November 12, pp. 55–76.

Gorski, R. A. 1974. The neuroendocrine regulation of sexual behavior. In *Advances in Psychobiology*, Vol. 2, edited by G. Newton and A. Riesen. New York: Wiley.

Grayson, J. 1960. *Nerves, Brain, and Man*. New York: Taplinger.

Great Britain, Home Office, Drug Branch. 1974. *United Kingdom Statistics on Drug Addiction and Criminal Offences Involving Drugs*. London: H.M.S.O.

Great Britain, Ministry of Health, Committee on Morphine and Heroin Addiction. 1926. *Report*. London: H.M.S.O.

Grinker, R. R. 1937. *Neurology*. Springfield, Ill.: Thomas.

Groh, G., and Lemieux, M. 1968. The effect of LSD-25 on spider web formation. *Int. J. Addict.* 3:41–53.

Grossman, W. 1969. Adverse reactions associated with cannabis products in India. *Ann. Int. Med.* 70:529–533.

Gupta, S., *et al.* 1974. Impairment of rosette-forming T-lymphocytes in chronic marihuana smokers. *N. Engl. J. Med.* 291:874–877.

Harbison, R. D., and Mantilla-Plata, B. 1972. Prenatal toxicity, maternal distribution, and placental transfer of tetrahydrocannabinol. *J. Pharmacol. Exp. Ther.* 180:446–453.

Harmon, J. H., and Aliapoulios, M. A. 1972. Gynecomastia in marijuana users. *N. Engl. J. Med.* 287:936.

Harney, M. 1964. Trial and failure of the ambulatory treatment of (opiate) drug addiction in the United States. *Bull. Narc. (U.N.)* 16(2):29–40.

Heath, R. G. 1954. Definition of the septal region. In *Studies in Schizophrenia*, edited by R. G. Heath. Cambridge, Mass.: Harvard University Press.

    1964. Pleasure response of human subjects to direct stimulation of the brain: physiologic and psychodynamic considerations. In *The Role of Pleasure in Behavior*, edited by R. G. Heath. New York: Harper & Row.

    1972*a*. Marijuana: Effects on deep and surface electroencephalograms of man. *Arch. Gen. Psychiatry* 26:577–584.

    1972*b*. Pleasure and brain activity in man. *J. Nerv. Ment. Dis.* 154:3–18

    1973. Marijuana: Effects on deep and surface electroencephalograms of rhesus monkeys. *Neuropharmacology* 12:1–14.

    1976. Cannabis sativa derivatives: Effects on brain function of mankeys. In *Marihuana: Chemistry, Biochemistry, and Cellular Effects*, edited by G. G. Nahas *et al.* New York: Springer-Verlag.

Heath, R. G. (ed.). 1964. *The Role of Pleasure in Behavior: A Symposium by Twenty-Two Authors.* New York: Harper & Row.

Heath, R. G., and Gallant, D. M. 1964. Activity of the human brain during emotional thought. In *The Role of Pleasure in Behavior*, edited by R. G. Heath. New York: Harper & Row.

Heath, R. G., and Mickle, W. A. 1960. Evaluation of seven years' experience with depth electrode studies in human patients. In *Electrical Studies on the Unanesthetized Brain*, edited by E. R. Ramey and D. S. O'Doherty. New York: Harper & Row.

Hembree, W. C., *et al.* 1976. Marihuana effects upon human gondal function. In *Marihuana: Chemistry, Biochemistry, and Cellular Effects*, edited by G. G. Nahas *et al.* New York: Springer-Verlag.

Henderson, A. H., and Pubsley, D. J. 1968. Collapse after intravenous injection of hashish. *Br. Med. J.* 3:229–230

Henderson, R. L., and Tennant, F. S. 1972. Respiratory manifestations of hashish smoking. *Arch. Otolaryngol.* 95:248–251.

Herbst, A. L. *et al.* 1972. Clear-cell adenocarcinoma of the genital tract in young females. *N. Engl. J. Med.* 287:1259.

Hill, N. (ed.). 1971. *Marijuana: Teenage Killer.* New York: Popular Library.

Hockman, C. H., *et al.* 1971. Electroencephalographic and behavioral alterations produced by delta-9-THC. *Science* 172:968–970.

Hope, A., *et al.* 1971. The brain. I. *Life*, October 1, pp. 45–59.

Hunt, W. A. (ed.). 1970. *Learning Mechanisms in Smoking.* Chicago: Aldine.

Huot, J. 1976. Cellular alterations induced in vitro by delta-9-tetrahydrocannabinol: Effects on cell proliferation, nucleic acids, and plasma cell membrane ATPase. In *Marihuana: Chemistry, Biochemistry, and Cellular Effects*, edited by G. G. Nahas *et al.* New York: Springer-Verlag.

Indian Hemp Drugs Commission. 1894. *Report of the . . . Commission, 1893–94.* Reprinted as *Marijuana: Report of the . . . Commission, 1893–1894.* Introduction and Glossary by John Kaplan. Silver Springs, Md.: Jefferson, 1969.

Ingvar, D. H., and Risberg, J. R. 1967. Increase of regional cerebral blood flow during mental effort in normals and in patients with focal brain disorders. *Exp. Brain Res.* 3:195–211.

Iversen, S., and Iversen, L. 1975. *Behavioral Pharmacology.* New York: Oxford University Press.

Iversen, S., and Weiskrantz, L. 1970. An investigation of a possible memory defect produced by inferotemporal lesions in the baboon. *Neuropsychologia* 8:21–36.

Jacobson, E. 1970. *Modern Treatment of Tense Patients.* Springfield, Ill.: Thomas.

James, I. 1969. Delinquency and heroin addiction in Britain. *Br. J. Criminol.* 9(2):108–124.

Jasinski, D.R., *et al.* 1971. Review of the effects in man of marijuana and tetrahydrocannabinols on subjective state and physiologic functioning. *Ann. N.Y. Acad. Sci.* 191:196–205.

Johnson, B. D. 1975. Interpreting official British statistics on addiction. *Int. J. Addict.* 10:557–587.

Jones, H. B. 1950. Respiratory system: Nitrogen elimination. In *Medical Physics*, Vol. 2, edited by O. Glasser. Chicago: Year Book.

1951. Molecular exchange and blood perfusion through tissue regions. In *Advances in Biological and Medical Physics*, Vol. 2, edited by J. H. Lawrence and J. G. Hamilton. New York: Academic Press.

1971. The deception of drugs. *Clin. Toxicol.* 4:129–136.

1972. A report on drug abuse in the armed forces in Vietnam. *Med. Serv. Dig.* 23(8):25–36.

1974. The effects of sensual drugs on behavior: Clues to the function of the brain. In *Advances in Psychobiology*, Vol. 2, edited by G. Newton and A. H. Riesen. New York: Wiley.

1976. What the practicing physician should know about marijuana. *Private Practice*, January, pp. 34–40.

Jones, H. B., and Jones, H. 1972. A study of drug abuse and its prevention for the armed forces of the United States. Unpublished report to U.S. Department of Defense, Office of Alcohol and Drug Abuse.

Jones, K. L., *et al.* 1969. *Drugs and Alcohol.* New York: Harper & Row.

Jones, R., and Benowitz, N. 1976. The 30-day trip: clinical studies of cannabis tolerance and dependence. In *The Pharmacology of Marihuana*, edited by S. Szara and M. Braude. New York: Raven Press.

Judson, H. F. 1974. *Heroin Addiction in Britain: What Americans Can Learn from the English Experience.* New York: Harcourt.

Kalant, O. J. 1966. *The Amphetamines: Toxicity and Addiction.* Toronto: University of Toronto Press.

1968. *An Interim Guide to the Cannabis (Marijuana) Literature.* Bibliographic Series, No. 2. Toronto: Addiction Research Foundation.

Kandall, S. R., and Gartner, L. M. 1973. Delayed presentation of neonatal methadone withdrawal. *Pediatr. Res.* 7:320–392.

Kandel, D. 1973. Adolescent marijuana use: Role of parents and peers. *Science* 181:1067–1070.

Karlins, M., and Andrews, L. 1972. *Bio-feedback: Turning on the Power of Your Mind.* Philadelphia: Lippincott.

Kaymakçalan, S. 1972. Physiological and psychological dependence on THC in rhesus monkeys. In *Cannabis and Its Derivatives*, edited by W. D. M. Paton and J. Crown. London: Oxford University Press.

1973. Tolerance to and dependence on cannabis. *Bull. Narc.* (*U.N.*) 15(4):39–47.

Keeler, M. H., *et al.* 1968. Spontaneous recurrence of marihuana effect. *Am. J. Psychiatry* 125:384–386.

Kern, E., *et al.* 1971. The brain. II. The amazing cells that command our bodies. *Life*, October 22, pp. 42–64.

Keville, K. (ed.). 1971. *Where To Get Help for a Drug Problem.* Hauppauge, N.Y.: Award Books.

Kew, M. C., *et al.* 1969. Possible hepatotoxicity of cannabis. *Lancet* 1:578–579.

Kier, L. C. 1975. A simple method for the determination of the smoking of marijuana. In *Alcohol, Drugs, and Traffic Safety: Proceedings of the 6th International Conference on Alcohol, Drugs, and Traffic*

Safety, Toronto, September 8–13, 1974, edited by S. Israelstam and
S. Lambert. Toronto: Addiction Research Foundation of Ontario.

Kiloh, L. G., and Bell, D. S. (eds.). 1971. *Alcoholism and Drug Dependency*. London: Butterworth.

King, A. B., and Cowen, D. L. 1969. Effect of intravenous injection of
marihuana. *J.A.M.A.* 210:724–725.

King, A. B., *et al*. 1970. Intravenous injection of crude marihuana.
J.A.M.A. 214:1711.

Kiplinger, G. F., *et al*. 1971. Dose-response analysis of the effects of
tetrahydrocannabinol in man. *Clin. Pharmacol. Ther.* 12:650–657.

Klausner, H. A., and Dingell, J. V. 1971. The metabolism and excretion
of delta-9-tetrahydrocannabinol in the rat. *Life Sci*. 10(1):49–59.

Klein, A. W., *et al.*, 1971.*Marihuana and automobile crashes*. *J. Drug Issues* 1(1):18–26.

Kolansky, H. D., and Moore, W. T. 1971. Effects of marihuana on
adolescents and young adults. *J.A.M.A.* 216:486–492.

1972*a*. Clinical effects of marihuana on the young. *J. Psychiatry*
10:55–67.

1972*b*. Toxic effects of chronic marihuana use. *J.A.M.A.* 222:35–41.

1975. Marihuana, can it hurt you? *J.A.M.A.* 232:923–924.

Kolb, D. A., and Boyatzis, R. E. 1970. Goal-setting and self-directed
behavior change. *Human Relations* 23:439–457.

Kolodny, R. C. 1975. Research issues in the study of marijuana and male
physiology in humans. In *Marijuana and Health Hazards*, edited by
J. R. Tinklenberg. New York: Academic Press.

Kolodny, R. C., *et al*. 1974. Depression of plasma testosterone levels
after chronic internal marijuana use. *N. Engl. J. Med.* 290:872–874

Kramer, M. 1956. *Public Health and Social Problems in the Use of Tranquilizing Drugs*. U.S. Department of Health, Education, and Welfare. Public Health Service Publication, No. 486. Washington:
G.P.O.

1967. Amphetamine abuse. *J.A.M.A.* 201:305–309.

Krause, S. O. 1958. Heroin addiction among pregnant women and their
newborn babies. *Am. J. Obstet. Gynecol.* 74:754–758.

Kreuz, D. S., and Axelrod, J. 1973. Delta-9-tetrahydrocannabinol: Localization in body fat. *Science* 179:391–393.

Landers, A. 1973. Ann Landers and her letters. *Berkeley Gazette* (Field
Newspaper Syndicate), June 4, p. 11.

Lassen, N. A. 1959. Cerebral blood blow and oxygen consumption in
man. *Physiol. Rev.* 39:183–238.

1974. Control of cerebral circulation in health and disease. *Circulation Res.* 34:749–760.

Lau, R. J., *et al*. 1976. Phytohemagglutinin-induced lymphocyte transformation in humans receiving delta-9-tetrahydrocannabinol. *Science* 192:805–807.

Lawrence, D. K., and Gill, E. W. 1975. The effects of delta-1-tetrahydrocannabinol and other cannabinoids on spin-labeled liposomes and their relationship to mechanisms of general anesthesia. *Mol. Pharmacol.* 11:595–602.

Lehmann, W. X. 1971. Doctor, what about marijuana? *Readers Digest*, April, pp. 169–176.

Lemberger, L., *et al.* 1970. Marihuana: Studies on the disposition and metabolism of delta-9-tetrahydrocannabinol in man. *Science* 170:1320–1322.

　　1971. Delta-9-THC metabolism and disposition in long term marihuana smokers. *Science* 173:72–74.

　　1972. 11-Hydroxy delta-9-tetrahydrocannabinol: Pharmacology, disposition and metabolism of a major metabolite of marihuana in man. *Science* 177:62–63.

Lemere, F. 1966. The danger of amphetamine dependency. *Am. J. Psychiatry* 123:5.

Lennard, H. L., *et al.* 1972. The methadone illusion. *Science* 176:881–884.

Leuchtenberger, C., and Leuchtenberger, R. 1971. Morphological and cytochemical effects of marijuana cigarette smoke on epithelioid cells of lung explants from mice. *Nature* 234:227–229.

Leuchtenberger, C., *et al.* 1976. Cytological and cytochemical effects of whole smoke and the gas vapour phase of marihuana cigarettes on growth and nuclear protein metabolism of cultured mammalian cells. In *Marihuana: Chemistry, Biochemistry, and Cellular Effects*, edited by G. G. Nahas *et al.* New York: Springer-Verlag.

Lewin, L. 1931. *Phantastica: Narcotic and Stimulating Drugs, Their Use and Abuse.* Translated from the 2nd German edition, 1924. Reprint. New York: Dutton, 1964.

Lewis, B. 1970. *The Sexual Power of Marijuana: An Intimate Report on 208 Adult Middle-Class Users.* New York: Wyden.

Lewis, E. 1973. A heroin maintenance program in the United States. *J.A.M.A.* 223:539–546.

Lomax, P. 1970. The effect of marihuana on pituitary-thyroid activity in the rat. *Agents Actions* 1:252–257.

Louria, D. B. 1968. *The Drug Scene.* New York: McGraw-Hill.

　　1971. *Overcoming Drugs.* New York: McGraw-Hill.

Ludwig, A., and Levine, J. 1965. Patterns of hallucinogenic drug abuse. *J.A.M.A.* 191:92–96.

Luthra, Y. K., *et al*. 1975. Differential neurochemistry and temporal pattern in rats treated orally with delta-9-tetrahydrocannabinol for periods up to six months. *Toxicol. Appl. Pharmacol.* 32:418–431.

Lynch, M. 1960. Brain lesions in chronic alcoholism. *Arch. Pathol.* 69:342–353.

McClelland, D. C. 1965. Toward a theory of motive acquisition. *Am. Psychol.* 20:321–333.

McCoy, A. M. 1972, *The Politics of Heroin in Southeast Asia*. New York: Harper and Row.

McEwen, B. S. 1975. The brain as a target organ of endocrine hormones. *Hosp. Practice* 10(5):95–104.

McGlothlin, W., *et al*. 1967. Long-lasting effects of LSD on normals. *Arch. Gen. Psychiatry* 17:521–532.

McIsaac, W. M., *et al*. 1971. Distribution of marihuana in monkey brain and concomitant behavioral effects. *Nature* 230:593–594.

McMillan, D. E., *et al*. 1970. Delta-9-trans-tetrahydrocannabinol in pigeons: Tolerance to the behavioral effects. *Science* 169:501.

Macey, R. I. 1968. *Human Physiology*. Englewood Cliffs, N.J.: Prentice-Hall.

Malcolm, A. I. 1975. *The Craving for the High*. New York: Simon & Schuster.

Manheimer, D., *et al*. 1969. Psychotherapeutic drugs: Use among adults in California. *Calif. Med*.109:445–451.

Mann, T. 1972. Drugs and male sexual function. *Res. Reprod.* 4(2):1–3.

Manno, J. E., *et al*. 1970. Comparative effects of smoking marijuana or placebo on human motor and mental performance. *Clin. Pharmacol. Ther.* 11:808–815.

Markam, J. M. 1972. What's all this talk of heroin maintenance? *New York Times Magazine*, July 2, p. 6.

Maugh, T. H. 1974*a*. Marihuana: Does it damage the brain? *Science* 185:775–776.

 1974*b*. Marihuana: The grass may no longer be greener. *Science* 185:683–685.

 1975. Marihuana: New support for immune and reproductive hazards *Science* 190:865–867.

 1976. Marihuana: A conversation with NIDA's Robert L. DuPont. *Science* 192:647–649.

Maurer, D. W., and Vogel, V. H. 1969. *Narcotics and Narcotic Addiction*. Springfield, Ill.: Thomas.

May, S., *et al*. 1975. Interrelationship between fatty liver, testicular atrophy, and alcohol consumption. Paper presented by L. H. Kuller,

American Public Health Association Meeting, November 18, 1975, Chicago.

Mechoulam, R. (ed.). 1973. *Marijuana: Chemistry, Pharmacology, Metabolism, and Clinical Effects*. New York: Academic Press.

Melges, F. T., *et al*. 1974. Temporal disorganization and delusional-like ideation: Processes induced by hashish and alcohol. *Arch. Gen. Psychiatry* 30:855–861.

Mellinger, G. D., *et al*. 1976. The amotivational syndrome and the college student. *Ann. N.Y. Acad. Sci*. In press.

Mendelson, J. H., *et al*. 1974a. Final report: Behavioral and biological concomitants of chronic marihuana use. Unpublished report supported by contract from the Department of the Army to the Alcohol and Drug Abuse Research Center, McLean Hospital, Belmont, Mass.

   1974b. Plasma testosterone levels before, during, and after chronic marihuana smoking. *N. Engl. J. Med*. 291:1051–1055.

Merry, J. 1967. Outpatient treatment of heroin addiction. *Lancet* 1:205–206.

Miliman, J. D., *et al*. 1976. The thought disorders of the cannabis syndrome. Paper presented at the National Drug Abuse Conference, March 29, 1976, New York.

Miller, L. L. (ed.). 1974. *Marijuana: Effects on Human Behavior*. New York: Academic Press.

Milstein, M., *et al*. 1974. Effects of opium alkaloids on mitosis and DNA synthesis. Abstract. *Pediatr. Res*. 8:118.

Mintz, J., *et al*. 1974. Sexual problems of heroin addicts. *Arch. Gen. Psychiatry* 31:700–703.

Miras, C. J. 1967. Marihuana and hashish. Paper presented at the Department of Pharmacology seminar, September 11, 1967, University of Calfornia, Los Angeles.

   1969. Experience with chronic hashish smokers. In *Drugs and Youth: Rutgers Symposium on Drug Abuse, 1968*, edited by J. R. Wittenborn *et al*. Springfield, Ill.: Thomas.

   1970. In a discussion on pharmacological aspects of marijuana use, Part 3, Discussion 3. In *The Botany and Chemistry of Cannabis*, edited by C. R. B. Joyce and S. H. Curry. London: Churchill.

   1972. Studies on the effects of chronic cannabis administration to man. In *Cannabis and Its Derivatives*, edited by W. D. M. Paton and J. Crown. London: Oxford University Press.

Mirin, S. M., *et al*. 1971. Casual versus heavy use of marijuana: A redefinition of the marijuana problem. *Am. J. Psychiatry* 127:1134–1140.

Moreau, J. J. 1845. *Hashish and Mental Illness*. Translated by G. J. Barnett; edited by H. Peters and G. G. Nahas. New York: Raven Press, 1973.

Morishima, A., *et al*. 1976*a*. Effects of marihuana smoking, cannabinoids and olivetol on replication of human lymphocytes: Formation of micronuclei. In *The Pharmacology of Marihuana*, edited by M. C. Braude and S. Szara. New York: Raven Press.

1976*b*. Errors of chromosome segregation induced by olivetol, a compound with the structure of C-ring common to the cannabinoids: Formation of bridges and multipolar divisions. In *Marihuana: Chemistry, Biochemistry, and Cellular Effects*, edited by G. G. Nahas *et al*. New York: Springer-Verlag.

Munson, A. E., *et al*. 1976. Effects of delta-9-tetrahydrocannabinol on the immune system. In *The Pharmacology of Marihuana*, edited by M. C. Braude and S. Szara. New York: Raven Press.

Murphree, H. B., *et al*. 1967. Electroencephalographic changes in man following smoking. *Ann. N.Y. Acad. Sci.* 142:245–260.

Musto, D. F. 1972. The city's heroin clinic: It was 1919. *New York Times*, June 6, p. 39M.

Nahas, G. G. 1973. *Marijuana: Deceptive Weed*. New York: Raven Press.

1975*a*. The patho-physiological effect of marijuana use in man. *Private Practice*, January, pp. 56–65.

1975*b*. When friends or patients ask about marijuana. *J.A.M.A.* 233:79–80.

1976. *Keep Off the Grass: A Scientist's Documented Account of Marijuana's Destructive Effects*. New York: Reader's Digest Press.

Nahas, G. G., and Greenwood, A. 1974. The first report of the National Commission on Marihuana (1972): Signal of misunderstanding or exercise in ambiguity? *Bull. N.Y. Acad. Med.* (2nd series) 50(1):55–75.

Nahas, G. G., *et al*. 1974. Inhibition of cellular mediated immunity in marijuana smokers. *Science* 183:419–420.

Nahas, G. G., *et al*. (eds.). 1976. *Marihuana: Chemistry, Biochemistry, and Cellular Effects*. New York : Springer-Verlag.

Nail, R. L. 1974. Motives for drug use among light and heavy users. *J. Nerv. Ment. Dis.* 159(2):131–136.

Negrete, J. C. 1973. Psychological adverse effects of cannabis smoking: A tentative classification. *Can. Med. Assoc. J.* 108:195–202.

Neu, R. L., *et al*. 1970. Delta-8 and delta-9-tetrahydrocannabinol: effects on cultured human leucocytes. *J. Clin. Pharmacol.* 10:228–230.

New York City Mayor's Committee on Marihuana. 1944. *Report on the*

Marihuana Problem in the City of New York. Lancaster, Pa.: Jacques Cottell Press.

New York Times Magazine, May 4, 1975. Letters to the editor, pp. 71–74.

Nichols, W., *et al*. 1974. Cytogenetic studies on human subjects receiving marihuana and delta-9 THC. *Mutation Res*. 26:413–417.

Nilsson, L., and Hydén, H. 1971. (Scanning electron microscopic photographs of the brain.) *Life*, October 22, pp. 42–52.

Olds, J. 1956. Pleasure centers in the brain. *Sci. Am.* 195(4):105–116.
   1958. Self-stimulation of the brain: Its use to study local effects on hunger, sex, and drugs. *Science* 127:315–325.

Olesen, J. 1971. Contralateral focal increase of cerebral blood flow in man during arm work. *Brain* 94:635–646.

Oswald, I., and Thacore, V. R. 1963. Amphetamine and phenmetrazine addiction: Physiological abnormalities in the abstinence syndrome. *Br. Med. J.* 2:427–431.

Patch, V. D. 1974. The dangers of diazepam, a street drug. *New Engl. J. Med.* 290:807.

Paton, W. D. M. 1968. Drug dependence: A socio-pharmacological assessment. *Adv. Sci.*, December, pp. 200–212.
   1969. A pharmacological approach to drug dependence and drug tolerance. In *Scientific Basis of Drug Dependence*, edited by H. Steinberg. London: Churchill.
   1972. Guide to drugs. 5. Cannabis. *Drugs and Society* 1(9):17–20.
   1973. Cannabis and its problems. *Proc. R. Soc. Med.* 66:718–721.
   1975. Pharmacology of marijuana. *Annu. Rev. Pharmacol.* 15:191–220.

Paton, W. D. M., and Crown, J. (eds.). 1972. *Cannabis and Its Derivatives: Pharmacology and Exerimental Psychology*. London: Oxford University Press.

Paton, W. D. M., and Pertwee, R. G. 1973a. The actions of cannabis in man. In *Marijuana: Chemistry, Pharmacology, Metabolism, and Clinical Effects*, edited by R. Mechoulam. New York: Academic Press.
   1973b. The pharmacology of cannabis in animals. In *Marijuana: Chemistry, Pharmacology, Metabolism, and Clinical Effects*, edited by R. Mechoulam. New York: Academic Press.

Paton, W. D. M., *et al*. 1972. The general pharmacology of cannabinoids. In *Cannabis and Its Derivatives*, edited by W. D. M. Paton and J. Crown. London: Oxford University Press.

Patrick, C. H. 1952. *Alcohol, Culture, and Society*. New York: AMS Press.

Payne, R. J., and Brand, S. N. 1975. The toxicity of intravenously used marihuana. *J.A.M.A.* 233:351–354.

Pellitier, K. R. 1975. Diagnosis, procedures and phenomenology of clinical biofeedback. Paper presented to Biofeedback Research Society, January 1975, Monterey, Cal.

Penfield, W., and Perot, P. 1963. The brain's record of auditory and visual experience. *Brain* 86:595–696.

Peterson, B. H., *et al.* 1974. Studies of the immune response in chronic marijuana smokers. *Pharmacologist* 16:259.

Pines, M. 1975. Speak memory: The riddle of recall and forgetfulness. *Saturday Review*, August 9, pp. 16–20.

Post, R. M. 1975. Cocaine psychoses: A continued model. *Am. J. Psychiatry* 132:225–231.

Post, R. M., and Kopanda, R. T. 1975. Cocaine, kindling, and reverse tolerance. *Lancet* 1:409–410.

Rajegowda, B. K., *et al.* 1972. Methadone withdrawal in newborn infants. *J. Pediatr. Res.* 81:532–534.

Renault, P. F., *et al.* 1971. Marijuana: Standardized smoke administration and dose effect curves on heart rate in humans. *Science* 174:589–591.

Robins, L. N. 1974. *The Vietnam Drug User Returns.* U.S. Executive Office of the President, Special Action Office for Drug Abuse Prevention. Special Action Office Monograph, Series A, No. 2. Washington: G.P.O.

Rodin, E. A., *et al.* 1970. The marijuana-induced "social high": Neurological and electroencephalographic concomitants. *J.A.M.A.* 213:1300–1302.

Roeder, F. D. 1973. Stereotaktische Therapie der Suchten. In *Vorbeugung und Behandlung bei Kriminellen und Süchtigen*, edited by G. Nass. Verlag Gesellschaft für vorbeugende Verbrechensbekämpfung in Kassel, Klinikstr, 7.

Roizin, L., *et al.* 1972. Methadone fatalities in heroin addicts. *Psychiatr. Q.* 46:393–410.

Rosenfeld, A., and Klivington, K. W. 1975. Inside the brain: The last great frontier. *Saturday Review*, August 9, pp. 13–15.

Rosenkrantz, H., *et al.* 1975. Oral delta-9-tetrahydrocannabinol toxicity in rats treated for periods up to six months. *Toxicol. Appl. Pharmacol.* 32:399–417.

Rosenthal, M. S. 1972. *Drugs, Parents, and Children.* Boston: Houghton Mifflin.

Rosenthal, T., *et al.* 1964. The development of narcotics addiction among the newborn. In *Drug Addiction in Youth*, edited by E. Harms. New York: Pergamon Press.

Rosenzweig, M., *et al*. 1975. Effect of enriched experience on recovery of rats from cortical lesions: Problem-solving scores and brain measures. *Neurosci. Abstracts* 1:508.

Rubin, V., and Comitas, L. 1972. *Effects of Chronic Smoking of Cannabis in Jamaica*. Report presented by the Research Institute for the Study of Man to the National Institute of Mental Health (Contract No. 42-70-97).

   1975. *Ganja in Jamaica: A Medical Anthropological Study of Chronic Marihuana Use*. The Hague: Mouton.

Russell, G. K. 1975. *Marijuana Today*. New York: Myrim Institute.

Saghir, M. T., *et al*. 1970. Homosexuality. IV. Psychiatric disorders and disability in the female homosexual. *Am. J. Psychiatry* 127:147–154.

San Francisco Chronicle. 1975. Science acquits pot of real harm. July 10, p. 36.

Scher, J. 1970. The marijuana habit. *J.A.M.A.* 214:1120.

Schwartz, G. E. 1972. Voluntary control of human cardiovascular integration and differentiation through feedback and reward. *Science* 175:90–93.

Schwarz, C. J. 1971. A toxic theory linking acute cannabis intoxication and regular use. Paper presented at the Western Institute of Drug Problems, August 7, 1971, University of Oregon, Portland.

Singh, J., *et al*. 1972. *Drug Addiction: Experimental Pharmacology*. Mount Kisco, N.Y.: Futura.

Smiley, A., *et al*. 1975. The combined effects of alcohol and common psychoactive drugs. II. Field studies with an instrumented automobile. In *Alcohol, Drugs, and Traffic Safety: Proceedings of the 6th International Conference on Alcohol, Drugs, and Traffic Safety, Toronto, September* 8–13, 1974, edited by S. Israelstam and S. Lambert. Toronto: Addiction Research Foundation of Ontario.

Smythies, J. 1970. *Brain Mechanism and Behavior*. New York: Academic Press.

Solomon, D. 1966. *The Marijuana Papers*. Indianapolis: Bobbs-Merrill.

Solomon, J., *et al*. 1976. Uterotrophic effect of delta-9-tetrahydrocannabinol in ovariectomized rats. *Science* 192:559–561.

Soueif, M. I. 1967. Hashish consumption in Egypt. *Bull. Narc. (U.N.)* 19(2):1–12.

   1971. The use of cannabis in Egypt: A behavioral study, *Bull. Narc. (U.N.)* 23(4):17–28.

   1973. Cannabis idealogy: A study of opinions and beliefs centering around cannabis consumption. *Bull. Narc. (U.N.)* 25(4):33–38.

1976*a*. Casting light on cannabis-type dependence: The psychology of chronic heavy taking. *Ann. N.Y. Acad. Sci.* In press.

1976*b*. The differential association between chronic cannabism and psychological function deficits. *Ann. N.Y. Acad. Sci.* In press.

Spear, H. B. 1969. The growth of heroin addiction in the United Kingdom. *Br. J. Addict.* 64:245–255.

Sperry, R. W. 1975. Left brain, right brain. *Saturday Review*, August 9, pp. 30–33.

Stanton, M. D. 1973. Marijuana flashbacks. *Am. J. Psychiatry* 130:1399–1400.

Stearn, J. 1969. *The Seekers*. Garden City, N. Y.: Doubleday.

Stefanis, C. N., and Issidorides, M. R. 1976. Cellular effects of chronic cannabis use in man. In *Marihuana: Chemistry, Biochemistry, and Cellular Effects*, edited by G. G. Nash *et al*. New York: Springer-Verlag.

Steinberg, H. (ed.). 1969. *Scientific Basis of Drug Dependence: A Symposium*. Biological Council, Coordinating Committee for Symposia on Drug Action. New York: Grune & Stratton.

Stenchever, M. A., *et al*. 1974. Chromosome breakage in users of marijuana. *Am. J. Obstet. Gynecol.* 118:106–113.

1976. The effects of delta-8-tetrahydrocannabinol, delta-9-tetrahydrocannabinol, and crude marihuana on human cells in tissue culture. In *Marihuana: Chemistry, Biochemistry, and Cellular Effects*, edited by G. G. Nahas *et al*. New York: Springer-Verlag.

Stent, G. S. 1972. Cellular communication. *Sci. Am.* 227(3):6–12.

Sterling-Smith, R. S. 1975. Alcohol, marijuana and other drug patterns among operators involved in fatal motor vehicle accidents. In *Alcohol, Drugs, and Traffic Safety: Proceedings of the 6th International Conference on Alcohol, Drugs, and Traffic Safety, Toronto, September 8–13, 1974*, edited by S. Israelstam and S. Lambert. Toronto: Addiction Research Foundation of Ontario.

Stone, M. L., *et al*. 1971. Narcotic addiction in pregnancy. *Am. J. Obstet. Gynecol.* 10:716–723.

Talbott, J. A., and Teague, J. W. 1969. Marihuana psychosis: Acute toxic psychosis associated with the use of cannabis derivatives. *J.A.M.A.* 210:299–302.

Tart, C. T. 1970. Marijuana intoxication: Common experiences. *Nature* 226:701–704.

Taylor, W. J. 1975. Methadone maintenance. *Int. J. Clin. Pharmacol.* 12:33–45.

Tennant, F. S., and Groesbeck, C. J. 1972. Psychiatric effects of hashish. *Arch. Gen. Psychiatry* 27:133–138.

Tennant, F. S., *et al*. 1971. Medical manifestations associated with hashish. *J.A.M.A.* 216:1965–1969.

1972. Hashish bronchitis. *J.A.M.A.* 217:1706–1707.

Thacore, V. R. 1973. Bhang psychosis. *Br. J. Psychiatry* 123:225–229.

Thorburn, M. J. 1972. In vivo chromosome studies in cannabis users and controls. In *Effects of Chronic Smoking of Cannabis in Jamaica*, edited by V. Rubin and L. Comitas. Report presented by the Research Institute for the Study of Man to the National Institute of Mental Health (Contract No. 42-70-97).

Tinklenberg, J. R. (ed.). 1975. *Marihuana and Health Hazards*. New York: Academic Press.

Tinklenberg, J. R., *et al*. 1970. Marijuana and immediate memory, *Nature* 226:1171–1172.

Toronto Star. 1975. Ottawa won't legalize marijuana, La Londe says. February 22, pp. 3–4.

Ulett, J. A., and Itil, T. M. 1967. Quantitative electroencephalogram in smoking and smoking deprivation. *Science* 164:969–970.

Ungar, G. 1974. Molecular coding of memory. *Life Sci.* 14:595–604.

United Nations. 1961. *Conference for the Adoption of a Single Convention on Narcotic Drugs*. 2 vols. New York: United Nations.

U.S. Congress, Senate Committee on the Judiciary, Subcommittee to Investigate Administration of the Internal Security Act. 1972. *World Drug Traffic and Its Impact on U.S. Security*. 5 parts. 92nd Congress, 2nd session. Washington: G.P.O.

1973. *Hashish Smuggling and Passport Fraud: "The Brotherhood of Eternal Love."* Hearing, 93rd Congress, 1st session. Washington: G.P.O.

1974. *Marihuana-Hashish Epidemic and Its Impact on U.S. Security*. Hearings, 93rd Congress, 2nd session. Washington: G.P.O.

1975. *Marihuana-Hashish Epidemic and Its Impact on U.S. Security: The Continuing Escalation*. Hearings, 94th Congress, 1st session. Washington: G.P.O.

U.S. Department of Health, Education, and Welfare. 1971. *Marihuana and Health: 1st Annual Report to the U.S. Congress*. Washington: G.P.O.

1972. *Marihuana and Health: 2nd Annual Report to the U.S. Congress*. Washington: G.P.O.

1973. *Marihuana and Health: 3rd Annual Report to the U.S. Congress*. Washington: G.P.O.

1974. *Marihuana and Health: 4th Annual Report to the U.S. Congress*. Washington: G.P.O.

1975. *Marihuana and Health: 5th Annual Report to the U.S. Congress.* Washington: G.P.O.

U.S. Domestic Council Drug Abuse Task Force. 1975. *White Paper on Drug Abuse: A Report to the President.* Washington: G.P.O.

U.S. National Commission on Marihuana and Drug Abuse. 1972. *Marihuana: A Signal of Misunderstanding.* First report. Washington: G.P.O.

1972. *Marihuana: A Signal of Misunderstanding.* Appendix, the technical papers of the first report. 2 vols. Washington: G.P.O.

U.S. National Institute of Drug Abuse. 1975. *Summary of Client-Oriented Drug Abuse Information Reported by the Client-Oriented Data Acquisition Process (CODAP): National Level Quarterly Report for the period January 1, 1975, through March 31, 1975.* Washington: NIDA.

Valenstein, E. S. 1973. *Brain Control: A Critical Examination of Brain Stimulation and Psychosurgery.* New York: Wiley.

Vander, A., et al. 1970. *Human Physiology: The Mechanisms of Body Functions.* New York: McGraw-Hill.

Wallace, R. K., and Benson, H. 1972. The physiology of meditation. *Sci. Am.* 226:84–90.

Walter, J. A. 1971. Drugs and highway crashes: Can we separate facts from fancy. In *Alcoholism and Drug Dependency*, edited by L. G. Kiloh and D. S. Bell. London: Butterworth.

Walton, R. P. 1938. *Marihuana: America's New Drug Problem.* Philadelphia: Lippincott.

Weil, A. T., et al. 1968. Clinical and psychological effects of marihuana in man. *Science* 162:1234–1242.

Wender, P. 1973. Some speculations concerning a possible biochemical basis of minimal brain dysfunction. *Ann. N.Y. Acad. Sci.* 205:18–28.

Widroe, H. J. 1975. Increasing cerebral function in brain-damaged patients. In *Human Behavior and Brain Function*, edited by H. J. Widroe. Springfield, Ill.: Thomas.

Wieland, W. F., and Yunger, M. 1970. Sexual effects and side effects of heroin and methadone. In *Proceedings, Third National Conference on Methadone Treatment, November 14–16, 1970.* U.S. Public Health Service Publication, No. 2171. Washington: G.P.O.

Wikler, A. 1968. Diagnosis and treatment of drug dependency of the barbiturate type. *Am. J. Psychiatry* 125:758–765.

Wilkinson, I. 1969. Clinical studies on regional cerebral blood flow. *Br. J. Radiol.* 42:638.

Winick, C., and Kinsie, P. M. 1971. *The Lively Commerce: Prostitution in the United States*. Chicago: Quadrangle Books.

Wolstenholme, G. E. W., and Knight, J. (eds.). 1965. *Hashish: Its Chemistry and Pharmacology*. London: Churchill.

Zeidenberg, P. 1973. Psychopharmacological hazards of legalizing marijuana in the U.S. New York State District Branches, American Psychiatric Association. *Bulletin 16:2.*

Zeidenberg, P., *et al*. 1973. Effect of oral administration of delta-9-THC on memory, speech, and perception of thermal stimulation. *Compr. Psychiatry 14:*549–556.

Zelson, E., *et al*. 1973. Neonatal narcotic addiction: Comparative effects of maternal intake of heroin and methadone. *N. Engl. J. Med.* 289:1216–1220.

Zimmering, P., *et al*. 1952. Drug addiction in relation to problems of adolescence. *Am. J. Psychiatry* 109:272–278.

Zimmerman, A. M., and Zimmerman, S. B. 1976. The influence of marihuana on eukaryote cell growth and development. In *Marihuana: Chemistry, Biochemistry, and Cellular Effects*, edited by G. G. Nahas *et al*. New York: Springer-Verlag.

Name index

Figures followed by the letter n refer to footnotes of tables on those pages.

Subject index

Figures in bold-faced type refer to pages on which illustrations or tables occur.